QUICK WEIGHT LOSS STRATEGIES

Transform your body: Unleashed Rapid Weight Loss with Our Strategies

Lydia. A. Dickens

The information contained in this book is for educational and informational purposes only. It is not intended as a substitute for professional advice, diagnosis, or treatment. Always seek the advice of your physician, healthcare provider, or qualified professional with any questions you may have regarding a medical condition before embarking on any health-related programs

Table of Contents

INTRODUCTION

Welcome to the transformative journey of achieving rapid weight loss through our fast diet plan. If you are seeking a powerful and effective approach to shed those extra pounds and reclaiming control over your health and body, you've come to the right place.

This comprehensive program is designed to accelerate your weight loss journey, providing you with the tools, knowledge, and support necessary to achieve remarkable results in a short amount of time.

In today's fast-paced world, the desire for quick results is understandable. We understand that you are eager to see tangible changes, and our fast diet plan is specifically tailored to meet that need. However, it's important to remember that rapid weight loss is not simply about shedding numbers on a scale—it's about transforming your lifestyle, redefining your relationship with food, and nurturing your overall well-being.

Our approach combines science-backed principles, sound nutrition, and strategic dietary guidelines to create a fast diet plan that maximizes fat-burning, optimizes metabolism, and promotes sustainable weight loss. This is not a crash diet that leaves you feeling deprived or hungry. Instead, it is a carefully crafted program that focuses on nourishing your body with nutrient-dense foods while keeping you satisfied and energized.

We believe that knowledge is power, and throughout this journey, we will equip you with the information and understanding necessary to make informed choices about your diet and lifestyle. You will discover the secrets behind effective weight loss, learn how to create a calorie deficit and unlock the key to making healthier food choices without compromising on taste or enjoyment.

However, we also recognize that weight loss is a deeply personal and individual experience. Therefore, our fast diet plan is flexible, allowing you to adapt it to your unique needs, preferences, and circumstances. We encourage you to listen to your body, honor your progress, and make adjustments along the way to ensure long-term success.

As you embark on this transformative journey, be prepared to witness physical changes, a shift in mindset, increased self-confidence, and improved overall well-being. We are here to support you every step of the way, providing guidance, motivation, and practical tips to overcome challenges and celebrate your achievements.

CHAPTER 1

The Science of Weight Loss

Diet Quality: The quality of your diet matters for weight loss. Emphasizing nutrient-dense foods like fruits, vegetables, lean proteins, whole grains, and healthy fats can help you feel fuller, support overall health, and make it easier to maintain a caloric deficit.

Macronutrient Balance: Balancing your macronutrients—carbohydrates, proteins, and fats—can impact weight loss. Protein-rich diets may help preserve lean muscle mass and promote satiety. A moderate intake of healthy fats and complex carbohydrates can also contribute to overall satisfaction and energy levels.

Physical Activity: Regular exercise and physical activity play a crucial role in weight loss. Exercise increases energy expenditure, promotes muscle development, and can boost metabolism. Combining cardiovascular exercise with strength training yields the best results for both weight loss and overall health

Metabolism: Metabolism refers to the processes by which your body converts food into energy. It can vary between individuals due to factors such as age, genetics, body composition, and hormone levels. While metabolism influences weight loss, its impact is often overstated. Instead of focusing solely on metabolism, creating a sustainable caloric deficit is more effective.

Behavior Modification: Modifying behaviors around food and physical activity is key to successful and sustainable weight loss. This includes mindful eating, portion control, identifying triggers for overeating, managing stress and developing a positive relationship with food and your body.

Sleep and Stress: Adequate sleep and stress management are often overlooked but crucial for weight loss. Poor sleep and chronic stress can disrupt hormone levels, increase appetite, and lead to weight gain. Prioritizing sleep and adopting stress reduction techniques like meditation or exercise can support your weight loss journey.

Individual Variability: Every person's body is unique, and factors such as genetics, medical conditions, medications, and lifestyle differences can affect weight loss outcomes. Concentrating on personal advancement rather than comparing oneself to others is important. Keep in mind that weight loss should be pursued with an emphasis on overall health and well-being.

Consulting with healthcare professionals, such as registered dietitians or physicians, can provide personalized guidance tailored to your specific needs and goals.

Factors Affecting Weight Loss

Weight loss is influenced by a variety of factors that can impact an individual's ability to shed pounds effectively. While the primary principle of creating an energy deficit remains constant, understanding these factors allows for a more nuanced approach to weight loss strategies.

Here are some key factors that can affect weight loss outcomes:

Genetics: Genetic factors play a role in determining an individual's metabolism, body composition, and how the body responds to different dietary and exercise interventions. Certain individuals may possess a genetic inclination to store fat more readily or experience a slower metabolic rate, which can present additional difficulties in the process of weight loss However, genetics do not solely determine one's ability to lose weight, and lifestyle factors still play a significant role.

Metabolism: Metabolism refers to the chemical processes in the body that convert food into energy. The basal metabolic rate (BMR) is the number of calories the body needs to maintain basic bodily functions at rest. Some individuals may have a naturally higher BMR, allowing them to burn more calories at rest. On the other hand, a slower metabolism can make weight loss more difficult. However, factors such as age, body composition, and physical activity level also influence metabolism.

Hormones: Hormones play a crucial role in regulating appetite, metabolism, and fat storage. Hormonal imbalances, such as insulin resistance or thyroid disorders, can affect weight loss. For example, insulin resistance can make it more challenging to regulate blood sugar levels and may lead to increased fat storage. Consulting with a healthcare professional can help identify and address hormonal issues that may hinder weight loss progress.

Age: Age can impact weight loss due to changes in metabolism and hormone levels. As individuals age, their metabolism tends to slow down, resulting in a lower calorie requirement. Additionally, hormonal changes during menopause can affect weight distribution and make weight loss more challenging for women.

Lifestyle Factors: Various lifestyle factors can significantly impact weight loss outcomes. Sedentary habits, a lack of physical activity, poor sleep quality, high-stress levels, and unhealthy dietary patterns can hinder weight loss efforts. Incorporating regular exercise, managing stress, prioritizing sleep, and adopting a balanced, nutrient-dense diet is important for successful weight loss.

Medications: Certain medications, such as antidepressants, corticosteroids, and antipsychotics, may have side effects that can contribute to weight gain or make weight loss more challenging. If you suspect that your medication is affecting your weight, consult with your healthcare provider to explore alternative options or strategies to manage weight while on medication.

It's important to remember that while these factors can influence weight loss, they do not determine one's ability to achieve successful outcomes. With the right strategies, mindset, and support, individuals can overcome these challenges and achieve their weight-loss goals. Consulting with healthcare professionals, registered dietitians, or certified fitness experts can provide personalized guidance tailored to individual circumstances and optimize weight loss progress

13. Setting Realistic Goals

When embarking on a weight-loss journey, setting realistic goals is essential for long-term success and maintaining motivation. Unrealistic or overly ambitious goals can lead to frustration, disappointment, and a higher likelihood of giving up. Here are some key factors to consider when setting realistic weight-loss goals:

Before setting weight-loss goals, it's necessary to assess your current health condition. Consult with a healthcare professional to evaluate your overall health, body composition, and any potential underlying medical conditions that may impact your weight loss journey. Understanding your starting point will help you set realistic expectations and tailor your goals accordingly.

Consider a Healthy Rate of Weight Loss: A healthy and sustainable rate of weight loss is generally considered to be 0.5 to 2 pounds per week. Rapid weight loss may be initially appealing, but it's often not sustainable in the long run and can have negative health consequences. Set a goal that aligns with this range to ensure you're promoting healthy habits and maintaining muscle mass while losing fat.

Focus on Non-Scale Victories: While the number on the scale is a common way to measure progress, it's important to remember that weight loss encompasses more than just the digits. Incorporate non-scale victories into your goals, such as improved energy levels, increased strength, an enhanced mood, or better-fitting clothes. Celebrating these achievements can boost motivation and provide a broader perspective on your overall progress.

Consider Your Lifestyle and Preferences: Setting goals that align with your lifestyle and preferences is crucial for long-term adherence. Consider your daily routine, work commitments, social engagements, and personal preferences when designing your weight loss goals. Choose strategies and behaviors that you enjoy and can sustain in the long run, ensuring that your goals are compatible with your lifestyle.

Break Down Goals into Smaller Milestones: Rather than focusing solely on the ultimate weight loss goal, break it down into smaller, more achievable milestones. This not only makes the journey more manageable but also provides a sense of accomplishment along the way. Celebrate each milestone reached, as these small victories contribute to the overall progress and keep you motivated.

Be Flexible and Adapt: Remember that weight loss is not always linear, and there may be fluctuations along the way. Be open to adapting your goals as needed, based on your progress, feedback from healthcare professionals, and changes in circumstances. Flexibility allows for a more realistic and sustainable approach to weight loss.

Focus on Overall Health and Well-being: While weight loss is often a primary goal, prioritize overall health and well-being. Make sure your goals include behaviors that support your physical and mental health, such as regular physical activity, balanced nutrition, stress management, and self-care. A holistic approach to weight loss ensures that you're not solely focused on the numbers but are nurturing your overall well-being.

By setting realistic weight loss goals, you can create a roadmap for success and ensure a positive and sustainable weight loss journey. Remember to be patient, kind to yourself, and celebrate each step along the way. With dedication, consistency, and realistic expectations, you can achieve your weight loss goals and maintain a healthy lifestyle for the long term.

CHAPTER 2

Assessing Your Current State

When embarking on a weight-loss journey, setting realistic goals is essential for long-term success and maintaining motivation. Unrealistic or overly ambitious goals can lead to frustration, disappointment, and a higher likelihood of giving up. Here are some key factors to consider when setting realistic weight loss goals:

Start with a Health Assessment: Before setting weight loss goals, it's important to assess your current health status. Consult with a healthcare professional to evaluate your overall health, body composition, and any potential underlying medical conditions that may impact your weight loss journey. Understanding your starting point will help you set realistic expectations and tailor your goals accordingly.

Consider a Healthy Rate of Weight Loss: A healthy and sustainable rate of weight loss is generally considered to be 0.5 to 2 pounds per week. Rapid weight loss may be initially appealing, but it's often not sustainable in the long run and can have negative health consequences. Set a goal that aligns with this range to ensure you're promoting healthy habits and maintaining muscle mass while losing fat.

Focus on Non-Scale Victories: While the number on the scale is a common way to measure progress, it's important to remember that weight loss encompasses more than just the digits. Incorporate non-scale victories into your goals, such as improved energy levels, increased strength, an enhanced mood, or better-fitting clothes. Celebrating these achievements can boost motivation and provide a broader perspective on your overall progress.

Consider Your Lifestyle and Preferences: Setting goals that align with your lifestyle and preferences is crucial for long-term adherence. Consider your daily routine, work commitments, social engagements, and personal preferences when designing your weight loss goals. Choose strategies and behaviors that you enjoy and can sustain in the long run, ensuring that your goals are compatible with your lifestyle.

Be Flexible and Adapt: Remember that weight loss is not always linear, and there may be fluctuations along the way. Be open to adapting your goals as needed, based on your progress, feedback from healthcare professionals, and changes in circumstances. Flexibility allows for a more realistic and sustainable approach to weight loss.

Focus on Overall Health and Well-being: While weight loss is often a primary goal, prioritize overall health and well-being. Make sure your goals include behaviors that support your physical and mental health, such as regular physical activity, balanced nutrition, stress management, and self-care. A holistic approach to weight loss ensures that you're not solely focused on the numbers but are nurturing your overall well-being.

By setting realistic weight loss goals, you can create a roadmap for success and ensure a positive and sustainable weight loss journey. Remember to be patient, kind to yourself, and celebrate each step along the way. With dedication, consistency, and realistic expectations, you can achieve your weight loss goals and maintain a healthy lifestyle for the long term.

Before embarking on a weight loss journey, it is crucial to assess your current state of health and gather relevant information about your body and lifestyle. This assessment serves as a foundation for setting realistic goals and developing an effective weight loss plan. Here are some key areas to consider when assessing your current state:

Body Composition: Understanding your body composition goes beyond simply knowing your weight. Assessing your body fat percentage, muscle mass, and distribution of fat throughout your body provides a more comprehensive picture of your overall health. This can be done through methods such as body fat calipers, bioelectrical impedance analysis, or dual-energy X-ray absorptiometry (DEXA) scans. Knowing your body composition helps you set realistic goals and track progress accurately.

Health History: Take into account your medical history and any existing health conditions. Certain medical conditions, such as diabetes, cardiovascular disease, or thyroid disorders, can impact weight loss efforts and require specific considerations. Consult with your healthcare provider to identify any potential health risks or limitations and develop a weight loss plan that accommodates your specific needs.

Lifestyle Habits: Evaluate your current lifestyle habits, including dietary patterns, physical activity levels, sleep quality, and stress management. Are there any unhealthy habits that contribute to weight gain or hinder weight loss? Understanding these habits allows you to identify areas for improvement and make the necessary changes to support your weight loss journey.

Emotional and Mental Well-being: Consider your emotional and mental well-being as they play a significant role in weight management. Reflect on your relationship with food and your overall emotional well-being. Identifying any emotional triggers or underlying issues can help you develop strategies to address them and create a healthier mindset around food and weight loss.

Support System: Assess the level of support available to you. Having a strong support system, whether it's family, friends, or a weight loss group, can greatly enhance your chances of success. Consider who can provide encouragement, accountability, and guidance throughout your weight loss journey. If needed, seek professional support from registered dietitians, personal trainers, or therapists who specialize in weight management.

Goals and Motivation: Reflect on your personal motivations for wanting to lose weight. Clarify your goals and what you hope to achieve through weight loss. Are you primarily focused on improving your health, enhancing physical fitness, or boosting your self-confidence? Understanding your motivations helps you set meaningful goals that align with your values and aspirations.

By thoroughly assessing your current state, you gain valuable insights into your body, health, habits, and support systems. This information forms the basis for setting realistic goals and tailoring a weight loss plan that suits your unique circumstances. Remember to approach this assessment with honesty, self-compassion, and a commitment to long-term health and well-being

2 Body composition analysis is a valuable tool for assessing the proportions of fat, muscle, water, and other components that make up an individual's body. It provides a more comprehensive understanding of overall health and helps tailor specific interventions, such as weight loss or muscle gain programs. Here are some key aspects of body composition analysis:

Body Fat Percentage: Body fat percentage refers to the proportion of fat in relation to the total body weight. It is an important indicator of overall health, as excess body fat is associated with an increased risk of various health conditions, including heart disease, diabetes, and certain cancers. Body fat percentage can be assessed using methods such as skinfold calipers, bioelectrical impedance analysis, or more advanced techniques like DEXA scans.

Lean Muscle Mass: Lean muscle mass refers to the weight of all non-fat components in the body, including muscles, bones, organs, and fluids. Maintaining or increasing lean muscle mass is crucial for overall health, as it contributes to a higher metabolic rate, improved physical performance, and better body composition. Body composition analysis can help determine the amount of lean muscle mass and guide strategies to preserve or build it.

Fat Distribution: The distribution of body fat is also important when considering health risks. Fat stored around the abdominal area (visceral fat) is more closely linked to metabolic disorders and cardiovascular disease compared to fat stored in other areas of the body. Body composition analysis can provide insights into fat distribution patterns and help identify areas that may require targeted interventions.

Hydration Levels: Body composition analysis can assess hydration levels by measuring total body water. Adequate hydration is essential for optimal bodily functions and overall health. Dehydration can affect body composition readings and lead to inaccuracies. Maintaining proper hydration is important for accurate and meaningful body composition analysis.

Progress Tracking: Regular body composition analysis allows for tracking progress over time. It helps monitor changes in fat mass, muscle mass, and overall body composition as you engage in weight loss or fitness programs. By periodically assessing body composition, you can make necessary adjustments to your approach and ensure that weight loss efforts are resulting in the desired changes in body composition.

Body composition analysis provides a more comprehensive understanding of the body beyond simple weight measurements. It helps individuals set realistic goals, track progress accurately, and make informed decisions regarding their health and fitness journey. Consulting with professionals who specialize in body composition analysis, such as registered dietitians or certified trainers, can provide personalized insights and guidance to optimize body composition and overall well-being

1. Body Composition Analysis

Body composition analysis is a method of assessing the proportions of different components that make up a person's body, including fat, muscle, bones, and water. It provides valuable insights into overall health, fitness levels, and body composition changes. Here are some key points about body composition analysis:

Importance of Body Composition: Body composition analysis goes beyond traditional weight measurements by examining the distribution of weight in different body tissues. Understanding body composition is crucial because it helps evaluate the balance between fat and muscle mass, which has significant implications for health, physical performance, and overall body aesthetics.

Methods of Analysis: Various methods can be used to analyze body composition. Some common techniques include skinfold calipers, bioelectrical impedance analysis (BIA), dual-energy X-ray absorptiometry (DEXA), and air displacement plethysmography (ADP). Each method has its strengths and limitations in terms of accuracy, cost, accessibility, and level of detail provided.

Body Fat Percentage: One of the primary measurements obtained from body composition analysis is body fat percentage. It represents the proportion of body weight that is composed of fat. A high body fat percentage is associated with an increased risk of obesity-related health conditions, while a healthy range is typically linked to improved metabolic health and physical performance.

Lean Body Mass: Lean body mass refers to the weight of all non-fat components in the body, including muscles, bones, organs, and fluids. It plays a crucial role in maintaining a healthy metabolism, supporting physical activities, and achieving a desirable body composition. Tracking changes in lean body mass can provide valuable insights during weight loss or muscle-building efforts.

Fat Distribution: Body composition analysis can help assess the distribution of fat throughout the body. The location of fat deposits, such as visceral fat (around organs) versus subcutaneous fat (under the skin), can have different health implications. Excessive visceral fat is associated with a higher risk of chronic diseases, while subcutaneous fat distribution is typically less concerning.

Tracking Progress: Regular body composition analysis allows individuals to track their progress accurately. By periodically assessing body composition, one can monitor changes in fat mass, muscle mass, and overall body composition. This information helps guide adjustments to diet, exercise, and lifestyle habits to achieve desired body composition goals.

Individual Variations: It's important to recognize that body composition can vary greatly between individuals due to factors such as genetics, age, sex, and physical activity levels. It is more meaningful to track changes in an individual's own body composition over time than to make direct comparisons to others.

Body composition analysis provides a comprehensive view of the body's composition, helping individuals make informed decisions about their health, fitness, and weight management goals. Working with professionals who specialize in body composition analysis, such as registered dietitians, fitness trainers, or medical practitioners, can offer personalized guidance and support to optimize body composition and overall well-being

2.2 Health Assessment

A health assessment is a comprehensive evaluation of an individual's overall health status, including physical, mental, and emotional well-being. It involves gathering information about medical history, lifestyle habits, current symptoms, and any existing health conditions.

Conducting a health assessment is important to identify potential risks, detect underlying health issues, and develop appropriate strategies for maintaining or improving health. Here are some key aspects of a health assessment:

Medical History: Gathering information about past and present medical conditions, surgeries, allergies, medications, and family medical history helps healthcare professionals understand your health background and identify any potential risk factors or hereditary conditions.

Physical Examination: A physical examination involves assessing vital signs such as blood pressure, heart rate, respiratory rate, and body temperature. It may also include measurements such as height, weight, and body mass index (BMI). Physical examinations can detect signs of specific health conditions, provide a baseline for future comparisons, and help determine overall physical fitness.

Lifestyle Assessment: Evaluating lifestyle factors is important for understanding their impact on overall health. This includes assessing dietary patterns, physical activity levels, tobacco or alcohol use, sleep quality, stress levels, and occupational or environmental exposures. Lifestyle assessments help identify areas for improvement and guide recommendations for healthier habits.

Symptoms and Complaints: Discussing any current symptoms, discomfort, or health concerns is an essential part of a health assessment. Detailing symptoms, their duration, severity, and any associated factors can assist healthcare professionals in identifying potential causes and guiding further investigations or treatment.

Mental and Emotional Well-Being: Assessing mental and emotional health is crucial for a comprehensive health assessment. It involves evaluating mood, stress levels, sleep patterns, coping mechanisms, and any signs of anxiety, depression, or other mental health conditions. Identifying and addressing mental health concerns is vital for overall well-being.

Professional Guidance: Consulting with healthcare professionals, such as primary care physicians, registered dietitians, or mental health practitioners, ensures a thorough health assessment and appropriate guidance. They can provide personalized recommendations based on the assessment findings, help create a preventive care plan, and address any specific health concerns.

Regular health assessments are beneficial for maintaining optimal health, detecting potential health issues early, and developing strategies to promote well-being. They serve as a foundation for establishing health goals, making informed decisions about lifestyle changes, and seeking appropriate medical interventions when necessary. By actively participating in a health assessment, individuals can take charge of their health and work towards a healthier and more fulfilling life.

2.3 Identifying Habits and Triggers

When it comes to making positive changes in our lives, understanding our habits and triggers is crucial. Habits are the behaviors we engage in regularly, often on autopilot, while triggers are the cues or situations that prompt these habits. By identifying our habits and triggers, we can gain insight into our behaviors, make intentional choices, and effectively work towards our goals. Here are some steps to help identify habits and triggers:

Self-Reflection: Take time to reflect on your daily routines and behaviors. Consider activities such as eating, physical activity, screen time, and sleep. Notice patterns in your behavior and identify the habits that are present in your daily life. For example, do you tend to snack mindlessly while watching TV, or do you often skip breakfast in the morning?

Keep a Habit Journal: Start a habit journal to track your behaviors. Write down what you do, when you do it, and the circumstances surrounding the behavior. Be specific and detailed. For example, note the time, location, emotional state, and any notable events or people present. This will help you identify recurring patterns and potential triggers.

Identify Cues and Triggers: Pay attention to the cues or triggers that precede your habits. These can be internal (emotions, thoughts) or external (people, places, or specific events). For example, you might notice that feeling stressed at work triggers the habit of reaching for unhealthy snacks. By identifying these triggers, you can become more aware of their influence on your habits.

Emotional Awareness: Recognize the emotions associated with your habits. Sometimes we engage in certain behaviors to cope with stress, boredom, sadness, or other emotions. Emotional eating, for example, is a common habit triggered by negative emotions. Identifying these emotional triggers can help you find healthier alternatives to address those emotions.

Experiment and Observe: Make small changes to your routine and observe the impact on your habits and triggers. For example, if you usually grab a sugary snack when feeling tired in the afternoon, try replacing it with a healthier alternative like a piece of fruit or a handful of nuts. Observe how this change affects your habits, and note any differences in your behavior or emotions.

Seek Support: Share your journey with a supportive friend, family member, or professional. Discussing your habits and triggers with someone can provide fresh perspectives and help you gain further insights. They can also offer encouragement, accountability, and suggestions for positive changes.

Develop Replacement Habits: Once you have identified habits and triggers, work on developing alternative behaviors that align with your goals. Replace unhealthy habits with healthier ones that serve you better. For example, if stress triggers the habit of reaching for snacks, find alternative stress-relief strategies such as deep breathing exercises, going for a walk, or practicing mindfulness.

By identifying habits and triggers, you become more aware of your behaviors and gain greater control over them. This awareness allows you to make conscious choices and develop strategies to replace unhealthy habits with healthier ones. Remember that change takes time and effort, so be patient and kind to yourself throughout the process. With persistence and self-reflection, you can cultivate positive habits that support your well-being and help you reach your goals.

Chapter 3

Nutrition Basics for Weight Loss

In the context of weight loss, nutrition assumes a vital role. By adopting healthy eating habits and making informed food choices, you can create a calorie deficit, support your body's needs, and achieve sustainable weight loss. Here are a few fundamental principles to remember when it comes to nutrition

Calorie Balance: Weight loss occurs when you consume fewer calories than you burn. To create a calorie deficit, it's important to be mindful of portion sizes and choose foods that are lower in calories but still nutrient-dense. Focus on consuming whole, unprocessed foods such as fruits, vegetables, lean proteins, whole grains, and healthy fats while minimizing the intake of high-calorie, sugary, and fatty foods.

Macronutrients: Pay attention to the three macronutrients: carbohydrates, proteins, and fats Carbohydrates serve as a source of energy and should be obtained from whole grains, fruits, and vegetables. Include lean proteins like poultry, fish, tofu, legumes, and low-fat dairy products to support muscle maintenance and promote satiety. Healthy fats from sources like avocados, nuts, seeds, and olive oil are essential for nutrient absorption and overall health.

Portion Control: Exercise portion control to effectively manage your calorie intake. Use measuring cups, a food scale, or visual cues to understand appropriate portion sizes. Aim for balanced meals that include a mix of proteins, carbohydrates, and fats, and fill up on vegetables and fruits, which are lower in calories and rich in nutrients.

Nutrient Density: Choose foods that are nutrient-dense, meaning they provide a high amount of vitamins, minerals, and other essential nutrients relative to their calorie content. Vegetables, fruits, whole grains, lean proteins, and low-fat dairy products are excellent choices for weight loss as they offer a wealth of nutrients while being relatively low in calories.

Hydration: Ensure proper hydration by consuming an ample amount of water throughout the day. Water helps support digestion, aids in controlling appetite, and can prevent the consumption of excess calories from sugary beverages. Opt for water as your primary beverage and limit the intake of sugary drinks, sodas, and high-calorie beverages.

Mindful Eating: Engage in mindful eating by being attentive to your body's signals of hunger and fullness. Take your time during meals, savor every bite, and respond to your body's indications of satisfaction. Eating mindfully can help you recognize true hunger and prevent overeating.

Meal Planning and Preparation: Plan and prepare your meals in advance to support your weight loss goals. This allows you to make healthier choices, control portion sizes, and avoid relying on unhealthy fast food or takeout options. Dedicate time to meal planning, grocery shopping, and batch cooking to set yourself up for success.

Seek Professional Guidance: If you have specific dietary needs, or health concerns, or need guidance on creating a personalized meal plan, consult with a registered dietitian. They can provide expert advice, tailor recommendations to your individual needs, and support you in achieving your weight loss goals in a safe and sustainable manner.

Remember, successful weight loss is a journey that requires patience, consistency, and a focus on overall well-being. Adopting healthy nutrition habits and making gradual changes to your eating patterns can lead to long-term weight management and improved health.

3.1 Macronutrients and Their Importance

Macronutrients are the three major nutrients that provide energy and are essential for the proper functioning of the body. They include carbohydrates, proteins, and fats. Each macronutrient plays a unique role and has specific importance in supporting overall health and well-being. Here's a breakdown of macronutrients and their importance:

Carbohydrates:

Role: Carbohydrates serve as a source of energy and should be obtained from whole grains, fruits, and vegetables. They provide fuel for physical activity, brain function, and various metabolic processes.

Importance: Consuming adequate carbohydrates is crucial to maintaining energy levels, supporting exercise performance, and promoting optimal brain function. Carbohydrates also play a role in regulating blood sugar levels and preventing the breakdown of muscle tissue for energy.

Proteins:

Role: Proteins are the building blocks of the body and are necessary for the growth, repair, and maintenance of tissues, including muscles, organs, skin, and hair. They also play a role in enzyme production, immune function, and hormone synthesis.

Importance: Consuming enough protein is essential for muscle development, recovery after exercise, and the maintenance of lean body mass. Protein also helps promote satiety and can aid in weight management by reducing appetite and supporting a healthy metabolism.

Fats:

Role: Fats are a concentrated source of energy and provide essential fatty acids that the body cannot produce on its own. Fats also serve as a protective cushion for organs, help insulate the body, and assist in the absorption of fat-soluble vitamins.

Importance: Consuming healthy fats is vital for hormone production, brain function, and the absorption of fat-soluble vitamins (A, D, E, and K). Including sources of unsaturated fats, such as avocados, nuts, seeds, and olive oil, in the diet supports heart health and reduces the risk of chronic diseases.

It's important to note that each macronutrient provides a different number of calories per gram:

Carbohydrates: 4 calories per gram

Proteins: 4 calories per gram

Fat: 9 calories per gram

Finding the right balance of macronutrients in your diet is key to meeting your energy needs, supporting overall health, and achieving specific goals, such as weight loss, muscle gain, or athletic performance. The ideal ratio of macronutrients may vary depending on individual factors such as age, sex, activity level, and health status. Consulting with a registered dietitian can provide personalized guidance to help you optimize your macronutrient intake and meet your nutritional needs.

3.2 Portion Control and Serving Sizes

Portion control and understanding serving sizes are important aspects of maintaining a balanced diet. and healthy diet. It involves being mindful of the quantity of food you consume and ensuring that it aligns with your nutritional goals. Here's an overview of portion control and serving sizes:

Portion Control:

Choosing the right carbohydrates is essential for maintaining a healthy diet and supporting overall well-being. Carbohydrates are a crucial source of energy for the body, but not all carbs are created equal. By focusing on selecting the right carbohydrates, you can ensure optimal nutrition and promote good health.

Here are some guidelines for choosing the right carbohydrates:

Whole Grains:

Whole grains are an excellent choice as they retain the entire grain kernel, including the bran, germ, and endosperm. This provides a wealth of nutrients, including fiber, vitamins, minerals, and antioxidants.

Examples of whole grains include quinoa, brown rice, whole wheat, oats, barley, and buckwheat. Look for "100% whole grain" on the packaging to ensure you're getting the full nutritional benefits.

Whole grains supply long-lasting energy, support digestive well-being, and aid in maintaining stable blood sugar levels.

High-Fiber Foods:

Opt for carbohydrates that are high in fiber. Fiber is beneficial for digestion, helps control blood sugar levels, promotes safety, and supports weight management.

Include plenty of fruits, vegetables, legumes, and whole grains in your diet, as they are excellent sources of dietary fiber.

Aim for a variety of colorful fruits and vegetables to get different types of fiber and maximize nutritional benefits.

Low Glycemic Index (GI) Carbohydrates:

The glycemic index assesses the speed at which carbohydrates elevate blood sugar levels. Choosing carbohydrates with a lower glycemic index can help promote stable blood sugar levels and provide sustained energy.

Foods with a lower glycemic index include whole grains, legumes, most vegetables, and certain fruits like berries and apples.

Avoid or limit highly processed and refined carbohydrates with a high glycemic index, such as sugary drinks, white bread, white rice, and sugary snacks.

Moderation with Refined Carbohydrates:

Refined carbohydrates have been processed and stripped of their fiber and many nutrients. They tend to be higher on the glycemic index and can lead to spikes in blood sugar levels.

While it's best to limit refined carbohydrates, you don't need to eliminate them completely. Include them in moderation as part of a well-balanced diet

If you choose refined carbohydrates, opt for whole-grain versions when available, such as whole-wheat pasta or whole grain bread.

Portion Control:

Even when choosing healthier carbohydrates, portion control is crucial. Be mindful of your overall carbohydrate intake and consider your individual needs, activity level, and health goals.

Balance your carbohydrate intake with adequate protein, healthy fats, and a variety of vegetables to create balanced meals.

By focusing on whole grains, high-fiber foods, low GI carbohydrates, and practicing portion control, you can make informed choices about the carbohydrates you consume. Remember that individual needs and goals may vary, so it's essential to listen to your body and consult with a registered dietitian for personalized guidance on carbohydrate intake and overall nutrition

3.5 Healthy Fats for Weight Loss

Incorporating healthy fats into your diet can actually aid in weight loss and support overall health. Healthy fats provide a feeling of satiety, help regulate blood sugar levels, and support various bodily functions. Here are some examples of healthy fats that can be beneficial for weight loss:

Avocados:

Avocados are rich in monounsaturated fats, which are heart-healthy fats that promote satiety and help control appetite.

Additionally, they serve as a beneficial source of fiber, vitamins, and minerals.

Add slices of avocado to salads, sandwiches, or use it as a creamy topping for toast or wraps.

Nuts and Seeds:

Almonds, walnuts, chia seeds, flaxseeds, and hemp seeds are all nutritious sources of healthy fats, protein, and fiber.

They provide a satisfying crunch and can be sprinkled on salads, yogurt, or blended into smoothies for added texture and nutrients.

Be mindful of portion sizes when consuming nuts and seeds, as they are high in calories.

Olive Oil:

Olive oil is a staple in Mediterranean cuisine and contains monounsaturated fats, which have been linked to improved heart health and weight management.

Use olive oil as a dressing for salads, drizzle it over cooked vegetables, or use it for light sautéing.

Fatty Fish:

Fatty fish such as salmon, trout, sardines, and mackerel are excellent sources of omega-3 fatty acids.

Omega-3s are known to reduce inflammation, support brain health, and contribute to a healthy metabolism.

Strive to incorporate fatty fish into your eating regimen a minimum of two times per week.

Coconut Oil:

Coconut oil comprises medium-chain triglycerides (MCTs), which are readily digested and can serve as a rapid energy source.

Studies suggest that MCTs may increase feelings of fullness and potentially enhance calorie burning.

Use coconut oil sparingly for cooking or baking, keeping in mind that it is high in calories.

Nut Butter:

Natural nut butter, such as almond butter or peanut butter, offer healthy fats, protein, and fiber.

Opt for options that do not contain added sugars or hydrogenated oils

Enjoy nut butter in moderation as a spread on whole grain bread, as a topping for fruit, or as an ingredient in homemade energy balls or smoothies.

Remember that while incorporating healthy fats into your diet can support weight loss, portion control is still important. Fats are calorie-dense, so it's essential to consume them in moderation within the context of a balanced diet. Consult with a registered dietitian for personalized recommendations based on your specific dietary needs and weight loss goals.

3.6 Protein and Muscle Building

Protein plays a crucial role in muscle building and repair. When combined with regular strength training exercises, consuming an adequate amount of protein can help support muscle growth and recovery. Here's why protein is important for muscle building:

Muscle Protein Synthesis:

Protein is made up of amino acids, which are the building blocks of muscle. When you consume protein, your body breaks it down into amino acids, which are then used to repair and build new muscle fibers.

Muscle protein synthesis refers to the mechanism through which the body constructs fresh muscle proteins. Consuming protein-rich foods or supplements stimulates this process, promoting muscle growth and repair.

Muscle Recovery:

Intense exercise, especially strength training, causes microscopic damage to muscle fibers. Protein is necessary to repair this damage and rebuild stronger muscle tissue.

Consuming protein after workouts helps kick-start the recovery process, reducing muscle soreness and improving overall muscle function.

Increased Muscle Mass and Strength:

Adequate protein intake, in combination with strength training, can lead to increased muscle mass and strength.

Consuming protein throughout the day, particularly during workouts, helps provide a constant supply of amino acids for muscle repair and growth.

Thermic Effect of Protein:

Protein has a higher thermic effect compared to carbohydrates and fats, which means that it requires more energy to digest, absorb, and process.

This increased energy expenditure can slightly boost metabolism, potentially supporting weight management and body composition goals.

Safety and Weight Management:

Protein is known to be highly satiating, meaning it helps you feel full and satisfied after a meal.

Including protein-rich foods in your diet can help curb cravings and prevent overeating, supporting healthy weight management and body composition.

Protein Sources:

Good sources of protein include lean meats, poultry, fish, eggs, dairy products, legumes, tofu, tempeh, seitan, and plant-based protein powders.

Strive to include a diverse range of protein sources to ensure a comprehensive array of amino acids

To support muscle building, it's recommended to consume around 0.7 to 1 gram of protein per pound of body weight (or 1.6 to 2.2 grams per kilogram) per day, spread across meals and snacks. Timing protein intake around workouts, such as consuming a protein-rich meal or shake within an hour after exercise, can be beneficial.

However, it's important to note that individual protein needs may vary based on factors such as activity level, age, and overall health. Consulting with a registered dietitian or nutritionist can provide personalized recommendations based on your specific goals and circumstances.

3.7 Incorporating Nutrient-Dense Foods

Incorporating nutrient-dense foods into your diet is crucial for overall health and supporting your weight loss goals. Nutrient-dense foods are rich in vitamins, minerals, and other beneficial compounds while being relatively low in calories. Here are some tips for incorporating nutrient-dense foods into your meals:

Fruits and Vegetables:

Strive to occupy fifty percent of your plate with an assortment of vibrant fruits and vegetables.

Choose from a wide range of options to maximize the intake of different vitamins, minerals, and antioxidants.

Include both raw and cooked vegetables in your meals to benefit from their unique nutritional profiles.

Whole Grains:

Opt for whole grains such as quinoa, brown rice, whole wheat, oats, barley, and buckwheat.

Whole grains provide fiber, B vitamins, minerals, and other beneficial compounds.

Swap refined grains like white bread and white rice with whole grain alternatives for added nutritional value.

Lean Proteins:

Include lean sources of protein in your diet, such as skinless poultry, fish, lean cuts of meat, tofu, tempeh, legumes, and low-fat dairy products.

Protein-rich foods provide essential amino acids for muscle building and repair.

Healthy Fats:

Incorporate healthy fats, such as avocados, nuts, seeds, olive oil, and fatty fish like salmon or sardines.

These fats provide essential fatty acids and fat-soluble vitamins, which are important for various bodily functions.

Dairy or Dairy Alternatives:

Choose low-fat or non-fat dairy products or their alternatives, such as unsweetened almond milk or Greek yogurt.

These options are good sources of calcium, vitamin D, and protein.

Legumes and Beans:

Include legumes and beans like lentils, chickpeas, black beans, and kidney beans in your meals.

They are high in fiber, protein, and other nutrients while being low in fat.

Nuts and Seeds:

Enjoy small portions of nuts and seeds as snacks or add them to salads, yogurt, or stir-fries.

They offer beneficial fats, protein, and fiber, as well as an assortment of essential vitamins and minerals

Hydration:

Hydration is essential for overall health and aids in digestion, nutrient absorption, and maintaining optimal body functions.

Remember, creating a balanced and varied diet that includes a wide array of nutrient-dense foods is key. Be conscious of serving sizes and pay attention to your body's signals of hunger and fullness. Consulting with a registered dietitian or nutritionist can provide personalized guidance to help you incorporate nutrient-dense foods into your weight loss plan effectively.

Chapter 4

Designing Your Diet Plan

Designing a personalized diet plan is an important step toward achieving your weight loss goals. Here are some key factors to consider when designing your diet plan:

Caloric Deficit:

In order to achieve weight loss, it is necessary to create a caloric deficit by consuming fewer calories than your body expends.

Calculate your daily caloric needs based on factors such as age, gender, weight, activity level, and weight loss goals.

Strive for a moderate caloric deficit ranging from 500 to 1000 calories per day, as it promotes consistent and sustainable weight loss.

Macronutrient Balance:

Determine the optimal macronutrient balance for your diet plan.

A well-balanced approach generally includes adequate protein, moderate carbohydrates, and healthy fats.

Protein helps preserve muscle mass, carbohydrates provide energy, and fats support various bodily functions.

Consult with a registered dietitian to determine the appropriate macronutrient ratios based on your specific needs and preferences.

Portion Control:

Pay attention to portion sizes to manage calorie intake effectively.

Use measuring cups, a food scale, or visual cues to understand appropriate serving sizes for different food groups.

Exercise caution with portion sizes when dining out or consuming pre-packaged foods.

Meal Planning:

Plan your meals and snacks in advance to maintain a balanced and nutritious diet.

Include a variety of nutrient-dense foods to ensure you meet your nutritional needs.

Consider meal prepping to save time and make healthier choices throughout the week.

Food Choices:

Choose whole, unprocessed foods whenever possible.

Focus on lean proteins, whole grains, fruits, vegetables, legumes, and healthy fats.

Minimize the intake of sugary drinks, processed snacks, refined grains, and high-fat foods.

Mindful Eating:

Engage in mindful eating to cultivate a more wholesome connection with food. Attend to signals of hunger and fullness, consume meals at a leisurely pace, and relish each bite.

Avoid distractions while eating, such as watching TV or working on electronic devices.

Hydration:

Ensure proper hydration by regularly drinking water throughout the day.

Water helps with digestion, metabolism, and overall well-being.

Restrict the consumption of sugary beverages and alcoholic drinks, as they can contribute unnecessary calories to your diet.

Adaptation and Flexibility:

Be open to adjusting your diet plan as needed based on your progress and feedback from your body.

Everyone's body is unique, so it may take some trial and error to find the right approach for you.

Allow flexibility in your diet to accommodate special occasions or social events while staying mindful of portion sizes and overall goals.

Remember, it's essential to consult with a registered dietitian or nutritionist to create a personalized diet plan tailored to your specific needs, health conditions, and goals. They can provide expert guidance and support throughout your weight loss journey.

4.1 Determining Caloric Needs

Determining your caloric needs is an important step in designing an effective weight loss plan. Here are some methods you can use to estimate your daily caloric needs:

Basal Metabolic Rate (BMR):

Your BMR represents the number of calories your body needs to maintain basic bodily functions at rest.

Use an online BMR calculator that takes into account your age, gender, height, and weight to estimate your BMR.

This calculation provides a baseline estimate of your daily caloric needs.

Harris-Benedict Equation:

The Harris-Benedict equation is commonly used to estimate total daily energy expenditure (TDEE), which includes your BMR and activity level.

Calculate your Total Daily Energy Expenditure (TDEE) by multiplying your Basal Metabolic Rate (BMR) with an activity factor. The activity factor varies based on your level of physical activity:

For individuals with a sedentary lifestyle (little to no exercise), the Total Daily Energy Expenditure (TDEE) can be estimated by multiplying the Basal Metabolic Rate (BMR) by a factor of 1.2. For those who engage in light exercise or sports 1-3 days per week, the activity factor is 1.375. Moderately active individuals (3-5 days of moderate exercise/sports per week) have an activity factor of 1.55, while very active individuals (6-7 days of intense exercise/sports per week) have an activity factor of 1.725.

Extra active (very hard exercise/sports, physical job or 2x training): BMR x 1.9

Monitoring and Adjusting:

Use the estimated caloric needs as a starting point and monitor your progress.

If you're not seeing the desired weight loss, you may need to adjust your calorie intake.

Gradually reduce your caloric intake by 250-500 calories per day to create a safe and sustainable caloric deficit for weight loss.

Professional Guidance:

Consult with a registered dietitian or nutritionist who can provide personalized guidance based on your specific needs, goals, and any underlying health conditions.

They can conduct a comprehensive assessment and provide more accurate caloric recommendations tailored to your circumstances.

It's important to note that these estimations provide a starting point, and individual factors can influence your actual caloric needs. It's also crucial to prioritize the quality of your diet, focusing on nutrient-dense foods rather than solely counting calories. This ensures that you're nourishing your body with the necessary vitamins, minerals, and macronutrients while promoting sustainable weight loss.

4.2 Creating a Calorie Deficit

Establishing a negative energy balance, where calorie intake is lower than expenditure, is a crucial element in achieving weight loss. To achieve a calorie deficit, you need to consume fewer calories than your body needs for maintenance. Here are a few approaches to assist you in generating a calorie deficit:

Determine your daily caloric needs:

Use methods such as the Basal Metabolic Rate (BMR) or the Harris-Benedict equation to estimate your daily caloric needs.

This provides a baseline for the number of calories you require to maintain your current weight.

Set a realistic calorie deficit:

Aim to create a modest calorie deficit to promote sustainable weight loss.

Generally, a deficit of 500 to 1,000 calories per day can lead to a gradual and healthy weight loss of 1 to 2 pounds per week

Prioritize nutrient-dense foods:

Place emphasis on consuming foods that are nutrient-dense, containing abundant vitamins, minerals, and fiber.

Choose lean proteins, whole grains, fruits, vegetables, and healthy fats to help meet your nutritional needs while managing calories.

Reduce portion sizes:

Regulate the size of your portions to effectively manage your calorie intake.

Use measuring cups, a food scale, or visual cues to understand appropriate serving sizes for different food groups.

Increase physical activity:

Regular exercise helps increase calorie expenditure, contributing to a calorie deficit.

Incorporate both cardiovascular exercises (e.g., jogging, swimming, and cycling) and strength training to maximize calorie burn and preserve muscle mass.

Be mindful of liquid calories:

Be aware of the calories in sugary beverages, alcohol, and high-calorie coffee drinks.

Opt for water, unsweetened tea, or other low-calorie alternatives to quench your thirst.

Seek support and guidance:

Consider working with a registered dietitian or nutritionist who can provide personalized guidance and support in creating a calorie deficit that aligns with your goals and overall health.

Remember, it's essential to prioritize a balanced and sustainable approach to weight loss. Severe calorie restriction can be detrimental to your health and may lead to muscle loss and nutrient deficiencies. Aim for gradual, steady weight loss and focus on long-term lifestyle changes for sustainable results.

4.3 Meal Planning Strategies

Meal planning is an effective strategy for weight loss as it helps you make healthier food choices, control portion sizes, and stay on track with your calorie and nutrient goals. Here are some meal planning strategies to support your weight loss journey:

Set a schedule:

Designate a specific time each week for meal planning and grocery shopping.

Consistency and routine can make the process easier and more manageable.

Incorporate variety:

Incorporate a diverse range of fruits, vegetables, lean proteins, whole grains, and healthy fats into your meal plan.

Consider portion sizes:

Practice portion control to manage and regulate your calorie intake effectively.

Use measuring cups, a food scale, or visual cues to understand appropriate serving sizes for different food groups.

Prep ingredients in advance:

Chop vegetables, cook grains, and portion out proteins in advance to save time during the week.

Preparing ingredients ahead of time makes it easier to assemble meals quickly and reduces the reliance on unhealthy convenience foods.

Plan for snacks:

Include healthy snacks in your meal plan to prevent reaching for unhealthy options when hunger strikes.

Opt for nutrient-dense snacks like fresh fruits, Greek yogurt, nuts, or cut-up vegetables with hummus.

Grocery shop with a list:

Before you go grocery shopping, prepare a comprehensive shopping list that aligns with your meal plan.

Stick to the list to avoid impulse purchases of unhealthy items.

Stay flexible:

Be open to adjustments and changes in your meal plan as needed.

Life can be unpredictable, and flexibility is important for maintaining a sustainable approach to meal planning.

Remember, meal planning is a tool to support your weight loss goals, but it's essential to listen to your body's hunger and fullness cues. Adapt your meal plan as needed, and be kind to yourself throughout the process.

4.4 Balancing Macronutrients

Balancing macronutrients is crucial for a well-rounded and nutritious diet. Here are some tips to help you achieve a balanced intake of macronutrients:

Understand the macronutrients:

Macronutrients consist of carbohydrates, proteins, and fats.

Carbohydrates provide energy, proteins support muscle growth and repair, and fats are essential for various bodily functions.

Determine your macronutrient ratios

The ideal macronutrient ratio depends on factors such as your age, gender, activity level, and specific goals.

A general guideline is to aim for a balanced distribution of approximately 45-65% of calories from carbohydrates, 20-35% from fats, and 10-35% from proteins.

Focus on high-quality carbohydrates:

Choose complex carbohydrates like whole grains, legumes, fruits, and vegetables.

These foods provide fiber, vitamins, minerals, and sustained energy compared to refined carbohydrates.

Incorporate lean proteins:

Include lean sources of protein such as skinless poultry, fish, lean cuts of meat, tofu, tempeh, legumes, and low-fat dairy products.

These options offer high-quality protein with lower levels of saturated fat.

Choose healthy fats:

Incorporate healthy fats into your diet, such as avocados, nuts, seeds, olive oil, and fatty fish like salmon or sardines.

These fats provide essential fatty acids and fat-soluble vitamins.

Portion control:

Be mindful of portion sizes for each macronutrient group.

Use measuring tools or visual cues to ensure you're consuming appropriate portions.

Prioritize whole foods:

Emphasize whole, unprocessed foods in your diet.

These foods often contain a balanced combination of macronutrients along with additional beneficial compounds.

Seek professional guidance:

Consult with a registered dietitian or nutritionist to determine the optimal macronutrient ratios for your specific needs and goals.

They can provide personalized recommendations based on your health status and individual requirements.

Remember, balance and moderation are key. It's important to tailor your macronutrient intake to your specific needs and preferences while considering your overall health and well-being. Listening to your body and making adjustments as necessary will help you find the right balance of macronutrients for optimal nutrition and weight management.

4.5 Understanding Food Labels

Comprehending food labels is crucial for making well-informed decisions regarding the foods you consume. Here are some key points to help you understand food labels:

Serving Size:

Give careful attention to the specified serving size indicated on the label. It indicates the recommended amount for one serving of the product.

All other information on the label, including calorie and nutrient content, is based on this serving size.

Calories:

Look for the calorie content per serving. This information tells you how many calories you would consume by eating one serving of the food.

Nutrients:

Check the amounts of macronutrients (carbohydrates, proteins, and fats) listed on the label.

Be mindful of saturated and trans fats, added sugars, and sodium content, as excessive amounts of these can negatively impact your health.

% Daily Value (%DV):

The %DV indicates the percentage of the recommended daily intake of a particular nutrient that one serving of the food provides.

Aim for a lower %DV for nutrients like saturated fats, sodium, and added sugars, and a higher %DV for nutrients like fiber, vitamins, and minerals.

Ingredient List:

The ingredient list provides valuable information about the contents of the food product.

The ingredients are arranged in descending order of weight, meaning that the first few ingredients comprise the largest portion of the product.

Be cautious of foods with long ingredient lists or ingredients that are difficult to pronounce.

Allergen Information:

Food labels often highlight common allergens, such as nuts, dairy, wheat, soy, or shellfish.

If you have any food allergies or sensitivities, carefully read the allergen information to ensure the product is safe for you.

Health Claims:

Pay attention to any health claims made on the packaging, such as "low-fat," "high-fiber," or "reduced sodium."

Remember that these claims are regulated and should meet specific criteria set by the food regulatory authorities.

Comparing Products:

Use food labels to compare similar products and make healthier choices.

Consider factors like calorie content, nutrient composition, and ingredient quality when making comparisons.

Context and Individual Needs:

Remember that food labels provide general information, but individual nutritional needs may vary.

Consider your specific dietary goals, health conditions, and personal preferences when interpreting food labels.

By understanding food labels, you can make more informed decisions about the foods you consume, better manage your calorie and nutrient intake, and work towards a healthier diet.

Chapter 5

Meal Ideas and Recipes

Here are some meal ideas and recipes to inspire your weight loss journey:

Breakfast:

Veggie omelet: Beat eggs with chopped vegetables like spinach, bell peppers, and mushrooms. Cook in a non-stick pan and serve with a side of whole-grain toast.

Greek yogurt parfait: Layer Greek yogurt, fresh berries, and a sprinkle of granola for a protein-packed and satisfying breakfast.

Lunch:

Grilled chicken salad: Toss grilled chicken breast with mixed greens, cherry tomatoes, cucumbers, and a light vinaigrette dressing.

Quinoa and vegetable stir-fry: Sauté mixed vegetables like broccoli, carrots, and bell peppers with cooked quinoa and a splash of low-sodium soy sauce.

Dinner:

Baked salmon with roasted vegetables: Season salmon fillets with herbs and bake until flaky. Serve with a side of roasted Brussels sprouts, carrots, and sweet potatoes.

Turkey meatballs with zucchini noodles: Prepare lean turkey meatballs and serve them over spiralized zucchini noodles with marinara sauce.

Snacks:

Apple slices with almond butter: Enjoy crisp apple slices with a dollop of almond butter for a satisfying and nutritious snack.

Veggie sticks with hummus: Dip carrot, celery, and bell pepper stick into a portion-controlled serving of hummus.

Smoothies:

Green smoothie: Blend spinach, banana, almond milk, and a scoop of protein powder for a nutrient-rich and refreshing smoothie.

Berry protein smoothie: Combine mixed berries, Greek yogurt, almond milk, and a scoop of protein powder for a delicious and filling snack.

Healthy Desserts:

To create baked apples, remove the core and slice the apples, then sprinkle them with cinnamon. Continue baking the apples until they reach a soft and tender consistency. Serve them with a dollop of Greek yogurt or a sprinkling of chopped nuts.

Dark chocolate-covered strawberries: Dip fresh strawberries into melted dark chocolate for a guilt-free, antioxidant-rich treat.

Remember to customize these ideas to fit your dietary preferences and nutritional needs. Experiment with herbs, spices, and different cooking techniques to add flavor without excess calories. Additionally, consider consulting a registered dietitian or nutritionist for personalized meal plans and recipes tailored to your specific goals.

5.1 Breakfast Options for Weight Loss

When it comes to breakfast options for weight loss, it's important to choose meals that are nutritious, and satisfying, and promote healthy eating habits throughout the day. Here are some breakfast ideas to support your weight loss goals:

Overnight oats: Prepare a simple and filling breakfast by combining rolled oats, Greek yogurt, and your choice of milk (such as almond, soy, or skim milk) in a jar. Add toppings like fresh berries, nuts, and a drizzle of honey or maple syrup. Let it sit overnight in the refrigerator, and in the morning, you'll have a ready-to-eat, nutrient-packed meal.

Vegetable omelet: Whip up a protein-rich breakfast by making an omelet with egg whites or a combination of whole eggs and egg whites. Add a variety of sautéed vegetables like spinach, mushrooms, bell peppers, and onions. Top it off with a sprinkle of low-fat cheese for extra flavor.

Greek yogurt parfait: Layer Greek yogurt with fresh berries, sliced almonds or walnuts, and a sprinkle of granola or chia seeds. Greek yogurt is high in protein, which helps keep you feeling full, and the combination of toppings adds a satisfying crunch and natural sweetness.

Prepare a slice of whole grain bread by toasting it, then spread mashed avocado on top as a topping. Add a poached or boiled egg on top for a protein boost. Season with salt, pepper, and a squeeze of lemon juice or a sprinkle of red pepper flakes for added flavor.

Smoothies: Blend together a nutrient-packed smoothie using ingredients like spinach, kale, frozen berries, a scoop of protein powder, and unsweetened almond milk or water. You can also add a tablespoon of nut butter or Greek yogurt for extra creaminess and protein

Cottage cheese with fruit: Enjoy a serving of cottage cheese paired with sliced fruits like berries, peaches, or pineapple. Cottage cheese is a good source of protein and provides a satisfying texture when combined with the natural sweetness of fruits.

Whole grain cereal with milk and fruit: Choose a high-fiber, low-sugar whole grain cereal and enjoy it with your choice of milk (dairy or plant-based) and a handful of fresh berries or sliced bananas. Look for cereals with minimal added sugar and ingredients.

Remember, portion sizes and overall calorie intake are crucial for weight loss. Additionally, it is vital to pay attention to the signals of hunger and fullness that your body sends. Adjust these breakfast options based on your specific dietary needs and preferences, and consider working with a registered dietitian or nutritionist for personalized guidance.

5.2 Lunch and Dinner Recipes

Certainly! Here are two lunch and dinner recipes that are delicious and suitable for weight loss:

Lunch Recipe: Quinoa and Vegetable Stir-Fry

Ingredients:

1 cup cooked quinoa

1 tablespoon olive oil

1 small onion, thinly sliced

2 cloves garlic, minced

1 medium carrot, thinly sliced

1 red bell pepper, thinly sliced

1 cup broccoli florets

1 cup snap peas

2 tablespoons low-sodium soy sauce

1 tablespoon sesame oil

1 tablespoon rice vinegar

Optional toppings: chopped green onions, sesame seeds

Instructions:

Warm up olive oil in a spacious skillet or wok on medium heat.

Add onion and garlic, and sauté until fragrant and slightly softened.

Add carrots, bell peppers, broccoli, and snap peas to the skillet. Stir-fry for about 5-7 minutes or until the vegetables are tender-crisp.

In a small bowl, whisk together soy sauce, sesame oil, and rice vinegar.

Move the vegetables to one side of the skillet, creating space on the other side to add the cooked quinoa.

Pour the sauce over the quinoa and vegetables, then stir to combine everything.

Continue cooking for an additional 2-3 minutes until everything is heated through. Serve the stir-fry in bowls and, if desired, add a garnish of chopped green onions and sesame seeds.

Dinner Recipe: Grilled Lemon Herb Chicken with Roasted Vegetable

Ingredients:

4 boneless, skinless chicken breasts

2 lemons, juiced and zested

2 tablespoons olive oil

2 cloves garlic, minced

1 tablespoon chopped fresh herbs (such as rosemary, thyme, or basil)

Salt and pepper, to taste

2 cups mixed vegetables (such as broccoli, cauliflower, and cherry tomatoes)

Cooking spray

Instructions:

In a bowl, whisk together lemon juice, lemon zest, olive oil, minced garlic, chopped herbs, salt, and pepper.

Put the chicken breasts in a shallow dish and pour the marinade over them. Allow the chicken to marinate for a minimum of 30 minutes or a maximum of 2 hours in the refrigerator.

Preheat the grill to medium-high heat. Take the chicken out of the marinade and discard any surplus marinade.

Grill the chicken breasts for about 6-8 minutes per side, or until cooked through and the juices run clear. The duration of cooking may fluctuate depending on the thickness of the chicken breasts.

While the chicken is grilling, preheat the oven to 425°F (220°C).

Coat the assortment of vegetables with a light drizzle of olive oil, along with a sprinkle of salt and pepper. Spread them on a baking sheet lined with foil and lightly coated with cooking spray.

Roast the vegetables in the preheated oven for about 15-20 minutes or until tender and slightly browned.

Take the chicken off the grill and allow it to rest for a few minutes before slicing it.

Serve the grilled lemon herb chicken with a side of roasted vegetables.

Feel free to adjust the portion sizes and seasonings based on your preferences and dietary needs. Enjoy these flavorful and nutritious recipes as part of your weight loss journey!

5.3 Snacks and Healthy Treats

Certainly! Here are two snack and healthy treat ideas that you can enjoy while pursuing your weight loss goals:

Snack Idea: Greek Yogurt with Berries and Almonds

Ingredients:

1/2 cup plain Greek yogurt

A quarter cup of assorted berries, such as strawberries, blueberries, or raspberries

1 tablespoon sliced almonds

Instructions:

In a bowl, spoon the Greek yogurt.

Add a layer of mixed berries and sliced almonds on top of the yogurt

Mix everything together gently.

Enjoy this protein-rich and satisfying snack!

Healthy Treat: Dark Chocolate Energy Bites

Ingredients:

1 cup old-fashioned oats

1/2 cup almond butter

1/4 cup honey or maple syrup

1/4 cup dark chocolate chips

2 tablespoons chia seeds

2 tablespoons unsweetened shredded coconut (optional)

1 teaspoon vanilla extract

Pinch of salt

Instructions:

Combine all the ingredients in a mixing bowl and stir until thoroughly combined. Transfer the mixture to the refrigerator and let it chill for approximately 30 minutes to firm up. Once cooled, shape the mixture into small, bite-sized balls using your hands. Keep the energy bites in an airtight container in the refrigerator for up to a week. Enjoy these delightful and nourishing treats as a midday pick-me-up or after a workout. Remember to practice portion control, be mindful of your overall calorie intake, and pay attention to your body's hunger and fullness signals. This snack and treat suggestions provide a well-balanced array of nutrients while satisfying your cravings in a healthier manner. Indulge in them moderately as part of a balanced and diverse eating plan.

Hydrating Beverages:

Staying properly hydrated is vital for overall well-being and can also aid in weight loss endeavors. Here are two refreshing and low-calorie ideas for hydrating beverages:

Infused Water:

Ingredients:

1 liter of water

Sliced fruits (such as lemon, lime, orange, berries, or cucumber)

Incorporate fresh herbs such as mint, basil, or rosemary into your dishes.

In a mixing bowl, combine the water with the sliced fruits and fresh herbs. Allow the flavors to infuse for a few hours or overnight in the refrigerator. Serve the infused water chilled and enjoy its refreshing taste while staying hydrated.

Iced Herbal Tea:

Ingredients:

1-2 herbal tea bags of your choice (such as chamomile, peppermint, or hibiscus)

1 liter of water

Ice cubes

Brew the herbal tea bags in boiling water according to package instructions. Let the tea steep for the recommended time, then remove the tea bags and allow the tea to cool. Transfer the tea to a pitcher, add ice cubes, and stir. Serve the iced herbal tea cold and savor its soothing flavors as a hydrating beverage option.

Add your choice of sliced fruits and fresh herbs to the water.

Stir gently to combine.

Place the pitcher in the refrigerator and let it sit for at least an hour to allow the flavors to infuse into the water.

Serve the infused water over ice for a refreshing and hydrating drink. You can refill the pitcher with water a few times before replacing the fruits and herbs.

Herbal Iced Tea:

Ingredients:

2 tea bags of your favorite herbal tea (such as peppermint, chamomile, or hibiscus)

4 cups of water

Ice cubes

Optional: Fresh lemon or lime wedges for garnish

Instructions:

Heat the water in a kettle or saucepan until it reaches a boiling point.

Place the tea bags in a heatproof container or teapot.

Pour the boiling water over the tea bags and let them steep for about 5-10 minutes.

Remove the tea bags and allow the tea to cool to room temperature.

Once cooled, transfer the tea to a pitcher and refrigerate until chilled.

Serve the herbal iced tea over ice cubes with a fresh lemon or lime wedge for added flavor.

Both infused water and herbal iced tea provide a flavorful and hydrating alternative to sugary beverages. They can be enjoyed throughout the day to quench your thirst and promote proper hydration. Remember to limit or avoid adding sweeteners to keep the calorie count low. Drink plenty of hydrating beverages to support your weight loss journey while maintaining a healthy and well-hydrated body

5.5 Eating Out and Making Smart Choices

Eating out can be challenging when you're trying to make smart choices for weight loss, but it's definitely possible. Prepare in advance: Take the time to review the restaurant's menu online before heading out to dine.

This allows you to review the options and make a more informed decision ahead of time. Look for dishes that are lower in calories, high in protein, and include plenty of vegetables.

Control portion sizes: Restaurants often serve larger portions than you need. Consider splitting a meal with a friend or asking for a to-go box at the beginning of the meal and packing up half of your entree to take home. This helps you avoid overeating and allows you to enjoy the meal over multiple servings.

Choose lean protein: Opt for lean protein sources like grilled chicken, fish, or lean cuts of meat. These choices are generally lower in calories and saturated fats compared to fried or breaded options.

Load up on vegetables: Look for dishes that incorporate plenty of vegetables, either as sides or as main components. Vegetables are nutrient-dense, low in calories, and help you feel fuller for longer.

Be mindful of cooking methods: Choose dishes that are grilled, steamed, baked, or broiled instead of fried or sautéed. These methods typically involve less added fats and calories.

Watch the dressings and sauces: Salad dressings, marinades, and sauces can be high in calories and unhealthy fats. Opt for dressings on the side and use them sparingly, or ask for lighter options like vinaigrettes or salsa.

Control your sides: Instead of opting for fries or other fried sides, choose healthier options like steamed vegetables, a side salad, or a baked potato (without excessive toppings).

Hydrate wisely: Be mindful of your beverage choices. Opt for water, unsweetened iced tea, or sparkling water instead of sugary drinks or alcoholic beverages, which can add unnecessary calories.

Practice moderation: While it's important to make smart choices, it's also okay to indulge occasionally. If there's a specific dish you really want to try, consider sharing it with others or enjoying a smaller portion.

Remember, eating out should be an enjoyable experience. By making mindful choices and being aware of your portion sizes, you can still savor delicious meals while staying on track with your weight loss goals.

Chapter 6:

Incorporating Exercise

Incorporating exercise into your weight loss journey is essential for achieving your goals and maintaining a healthy lifestyle. Select activities that bring you pleasure and satisfaction: Find physical activities that you genuinely enjoy

Whether it's walking, cycling, dancing, swimming, or playing a sport, selecting activities that you find fun and engaging will make it easier to stick with them long term.

Start with small goals: Begin with realistic and achievable exercise goals. Set small milestones to gradually increase your activity level. For example, aim to walk for 20 minutes three times a week and gradually increase the duration or intensity as you become more comfortable.

Make it a habit: Incorporate exercise into your daily routine by scheduling dedicated time for it. Consider it an essential commitment to yourself that cannot be compromised. Consistency is key, so aim for at least 150 minutes of moderate-intensity aerobic activity or 75 minutes of vigorous-intensity aerobic activity per week, along with strength training exercises twice a week.

Find a workout buddy: Exercising with a friend or joining a fitness group can provide motivation, and accountability, and make workouts more enjoyable. Having a workout buddy can make the experience more social and help you stay committed to your exercise routine.

Keep your exercise routine interesting by incorporating different types of workouts to prevent monotony. Try different forms of exercise to target different muscle groups and keep your routine interesting. Incorporate activities such as strength training, cardio exercises, flexibility exercises, and interval training for a well-rounded fitness regimen.

Be attentive to the signals your body sends during and after exercise, and respond accordingly to ensure a safe and effective workout.

Regenerate response Gradually increase the intensity and duration of your workouts over time, but be mindful not to push yourself too hard or risk injury. If you experience pain or discomfort, consult a healthcare professional.

Set realistic goals: Set specific, measurable, and attainable fitness goals that align with your weight loss objectives. Whether it's increasing your strength, improving endurance, or participating in a fitness event, having goals to work towards can keep you motivated and focused.

Keep a log of your exercise sessions and monitor your progress to stay motivated and gauge your improvement over time. This can be as simple as using a fitness app, journaling, or using a fitness tracker. Seeing your improvement over time can boost your motivation and help you stay on track.

Always seek advice from a healthcare professional before embarking on a new exercise regimen, particularly if you have any pre-existing medical conditions. Gradually ramp up the intensity and duration of your workouts to minimize the risk of injury and give your body time to adjust and adapt. Find activities that you enjoy and make exercise a regular part of your weight loss journey for long-lasting success.

6.1 Exercise plays a fundamental role in the process of weight loss

Exercise plays an essential role in weight loss and overall well-being. Here are some key ways exercise contributes to weight loss:

Calorie burning: Engaging in physical activity increases your energy expenditure, helping you burn calories. Creating a calorie deficit, where you burn more calories than you consume, is a fundamental aspect of weight loss. Different types of exercises have varying calorie-burning potentials, with high-intensity exercises generally burning more calories in a shorter time.

Boosts metabolism: Regular exercise can increase your metabolic rate, both during and after your workout. Intense workouts, such as strength training and high-intensity interval training (HIIT), have been shown to elevate the metabolism for several hours after exercise. This means you continue to burn calories even when you're at rest, supporting weight loss efforts.

Preserves lean muscle mass: When losing weight, it's important to preserve muscle mass. Exercise, particularly resistance training, helps maintain and build muscle, which is metabolically active tissue. As you build more muscle mass, your body becomes more effective at burning calories, even when you're not actively exercising.

Enhances fat burning: Exercise stimulates the breakdown of stored body fat for energy. Aerobic exercises like jogging, swimming, or cycling, performed at a moderate intensity, can tap into fat stores and promote fat loss. Combining aerobic exercise with strength training further enhances fat burning and promotes a leaner physique.

Appetite regulation: Exercise can influence appetite hormones, leading to better appetite control. It has been found that regular physical activity can suppress hunger and reduce cravings, making it easier to adhere to a calorie-restricted diet and maintain a healthy eating pattern.

Improves overall well-being: Regular exercise has numerous benefits for mental and emotional well-being. It helps reduce stress, improves mood, enhances sleep quality, boosts energy levels, and increases self-confidence. When you feel good mentally, it can positively impact your motivation and commitment to your weight loss journey.

Sustainable weight maintenance: Beyond weight loss, incorporating exercise into your lifestyle is crucial for long-term weight maintenance. Regular physical activity helps prevent weight regain by supporting a healthy metabolism, preserving muscle mass, and promoting a balanced and active lifestyle.

It's important to note that while exercise is beneficial for weight loss, it should be combined with a balanced and nutritious diet. The most effective weight loss approach involves a combination of regular physical activity, healthy eating habits, and lifestyle modifications tailored to your individual needs. It is crucial to seek advice from a healthcare professional before initiating any new exercise regimen, particularly if you have any pre-existing health conditions.

6.2 Types of Exercise for Weight Loss

When it comes to weight loss, incorporating a variety of exercises can be beneficial to challenge your body and keep your workouts interesting. Here are some types of exercises that can aid in weight loss:

Cardiovascular exercises: Cardiovascular exercises, also known as aerobic exercises, are great for burning calories and increasing your heart rate. These exercises elevate your breathing and heart rate, promoting fat-burning and weight loss. Some examples include:

Running or jogging

Cycling

Swimming

Walking

Dancing

Jumping rope

High-intensity interval training (HIIT)

Kickboxing or aerobic classes

Strength training: While cardio exercises are effective for burning calories during the workout, strength training is essential for building muscle and boosting your metabolism. As you gain more muscle mass, your body becomes more efficient at burning calories even at rest. Strength training exercises include:

Weightlifting

Bodyweight exercises (push-ups, squats, lunges, etc.)

Resistance band exercises

Pilates

Yoga (some yoga styles focus on strength-building)

Circuit training: Circuit training combines cardiovascular exercises with strength training, providing a well-rounded workout. This helps keep your heart rate up, burns calories, and engages multiple muscle groups. You can create your own circuit or join circuit training classes at the gym.

High-intensity interval training (HIIT): HIIT workouts involve short bursts of intense exercises followed by brief periods of rest or active recovery. These workouts are time-efficient and highly effective for burning calories and increasing cardiovascular fitness. HIIT can be performed with various exercises like sprinting, burpees, mountain climbers, or kettlebell swings.

Sports and recreational activities: Engaging in sports and recreational activities is an enjoyable way to burn calories and stay active. Whether it's basketball, soccer, tennis, swimming, or hiking, participating in activities you love can help you stay motivated and make exercise a fun part of your routine.

Remember to choose activities that you enjoy and that fit your fitness level. Gradually increase the intensity and duration of your workouts over time to avoid overexertion or injury. Aim for a combination of cardiovascular exercises, strength training, and other activities to create a well-rounded fitness routine that supports your weight loss goals. It's always a good idea to consult with a healthcare professional or a certified fitness trainer to tailor an exercise plan to your specific needs and abilities.

6.3 Creating an Exercise Routine

Creating an exercise routine that suits your goals and fits into your lifestyle is essential for long-term success. Here's a step-by-step guide to help you create an effective exercise routine for weight loss:

Define your goals: Start by identifying your specific fitness and weight loss goals. Do you want to lose a certain amount of weight, improve cardiovascular fitness, build strength, or enhance overall health? Clear goals will guide your exercise choices and keep you focused.

Evaluate your existing level of fitness to establish your baseline and starting point. Consider factors such as your cardiovascular endurance, strength, flexibility, and any specific limitations or injuries you need to be mindful of. This assessment will help you choose appropriate exercises and set realistic expectations.

Determine your available time: Consider your daily schedule and identify windows of time when you can commit to regular exercise. Strive to engage in a minimum of 150 minutes per week of aerobic exercise at a moderate intensity, or 75 minutes per week of aerobic exercise at a vigorous intensity. Additionally, incorporate strength training exercises into your routine two or more days per week. Break down your exercise sessions into manageable chunks based on your availability.

Choose your exercise modalities: Select exercises that align with your goals and interests. Incorporate a variety of exercises into your routine, including cardiovascular activities, strength training exercises, and flexibility exercises. For cardiovascular fitness, options can include walking, running, cycling, swimming, or group fitness classes. It entails transitioning from one exercise to another with little to no rest in between. Flexibility exercises like yoga or stretching can improve mobility and aid recovery.

Plan your routine: Map out your exercise routine for the week. Determine which days you'll dedicate to cardiovascular exercises, strength training, and flexibility work. Balance high-intensity workouts with lower-intensity or rest days to allow for recovery. Be flexible and adjust your routine as needed based on your progress and personal preferences.

Start slowly and progress gradually: Begin with lighter intensities and shorter durations if you're new to exercise or returning after a break. Gradually increase the duration, intensity, or frequency of your workouts over time as your fitness improves. This progressive approach helps prevent injuries and ensures continued progress.

Mix up your workouts: Avoid boredom and keep your body challenged by incorporating a variety of exercises. Alternate between different forms of cardiovascular activities, try new strength training exercises, or experiment with different fitness classes. This variety keeps your workouts engaging and prevents plateaus.

Track your progress: Keep a record of your workouts, including the exercises performed, duration, intensity, and any achievements or milestones reached. This helps you monitor your progress, stay motivated, and make adjustments to your routine if needed.

Pay close attention to the signals your body sends during and after exercise. Take note of any feelings of fatigue, pain, or discomfort, and respond accordingly by adjusting your workout or giving yourself adequate rest. It's important to rest and recover adequately to prevent overtraining and injuries. Remember that rest and recovery are integral parts of an effective exercise routine.

Maintain your motivation by discovering strategies that keep you inspired and committed. Set rewards for reaching milestones, find a workout buddy or join fitness communities for support, or consider working with a personal trainer or coach to keep you on track.

Remember, consistency is key. Stick to your exercise routine as much as possible, even on days when motivation is low. By creating a well-rounded and sustainable exercise routine, you'll not only support your weight loss goals but also improve your overall health and well-being.

6.4 Strength Training and Cardiovascular Exercise

Strength training and cardiovascular exercise are two essential components of a well-rounded fitness routine. Combining these two types of exercise can maximize your weight loss efforts, improve overall fitness, and promote a healthy body composition.

Here's an overview of the benefits and recommendations for incorporating both strength training and cardiovascular exercise into your routine:

Increases strength and endurance: Regular strength training improves muscular strength and endurance, allowing you to perform daily activities more efficiently and with less fatigue. It also helps prevent age-related muscle loss, maintaining functional independence as you age.

Enhances body composition: As you build muscle through strength training, you'll experience positive changes in body composition. While the number on the scale may not change significantly, you'll likely notice a reduction in body fat and a more toned appearance

Increases bone density: Strength training promotes bone health and helps prevent conditions like osteoporosis. Weight-bearing exercises, such as lifting weights or performing resistance exercises, put stress on the bones, stimulating them to become stronger and denser.

Supports joint stability and injury prevention: Strengthening the muscles around your joints improves joint stability and reduces the risk of injury. Strong muscles provide support and protection to your joints during physical activities and daily movements.

Cardiovascular Exercise:

Burns calories and promotes weight loss: Cardiovascular exercises elevate your heart rate and increase calorie expenditure. Engaging in activities like running, cycling, swimming, or aerobic classes can help create a calorie deficit, leading to weight loss

Improves cardiovascular health: Regular cardiovascular exercise strengthens your heart, improves blood circulation, and increases lung capacity. This lowers the risk of heart disease, high blood pressure, and other cardiovascular conditions.

Enhances endurance and stamina: Cardiovascular exercise improves your body's ability to deliver oxygen and nutrients to your muscles, enhancing overall endurance and stamina. This allows you to engage in physical activities for longer periods without feeling fatigued.

Reduces stress and improves mood: Cardiovascular exercise stimulates the release of endorphins, also known as "feel-good" hormones. This can boost your mood, reduce stress, and promote mental well-being.

Supports overall fitness: Cardiovascular exercise improves overall physical fitness and performance. It increases your energy levels, enhances respiratory function, and improves your body's efficiency in utilizing oxygen.

6.5 Staying Active Throughout the Day

Staying active throughout the day is just as important as dedicated exercise sessions for maintaining overall health and supporting weight loss efforts. Here are some actionable suggestions to assist you in integrating more physical activity into your daily schedule:

Take regular breaks: Whether you're working at a desk or engaged in other sedentary activities, make it a habit to take regular breaks. Set a timer or use reminder apps to prompt you to stand up, stretch, and move around every hour. Even a short walk around the office or your home can make a difference.

Walk whenever possible: Opt for walking instead of driving or taking the elevator whenever feasible. Choose to walk short distances, such as to the grocery store or to nearby destinations. If you use public transportation, consider getting off one stop earlier and walking the rest of the way.

Incorporate movement into daily tasks: Find ways to make your everyday tasks more active. For example, instead of using a remote control, here are some practical strategies to incorporate additional movement into your everyday life:

Instead of using a remote control, manually change the TV channel.

Opt for a standing desk or engage in activities like taking phone calls while standing and walking around the room.

Whenever feasible, choose the stairs over the elevator to increase your physical activity.

Engage in active hobbies: Pursue hobbies that require physical activity, such as gardening, dancing, swimming, or playing a sport. These activities not only keep you active but also provide enjoyment and fulfillment.

Set reminders for mini workouts: Incorporate short bursts of exercise throughout the day. Set reminders on your phone or computer to do quick exercises like squats, lunges, push-ups, or jumping jacks. These mini-workouts can be done anywhere, even in the comfort of your own home or office space.

Stand and move during screen time: If you spend a lot of time watching TV or using electronic devices, make an effort to stand up and move during commercial breaks or every half an hour. Do some stretching, march in place, or perform simple exercises to keep your body active.

Schedule active breaks: Plan intentional breaks during your workday or daily routine to engage in physical activity. This could be going for a brisk walk during lunchtime, doing a quick workout routine, or participating in a fitness class. Treat these breaks as essential appointments and prioritize them in your schedule

Involve others: Make staying active a social activity by involving friends, family, or coworkers. Plan active outings or activities together, such as hiking, biking, or participating in group exercise classes. Having a support system and shared accountability can make it more enjoyable and increase adherence.

Track your steps: Consider using a fitness tracker or smartphone app to monitor your daily step count. Set a goal to increase your steps gradually over time and challenge yourself to meet or exceed your target. This can serve as a motivating factor and help you stay consistent with staying active.

Remember, every bit of movement counts. Incorporating more activity throughout your day not only contributes to burning extra calories but also improves circulation, boosts energy levels, and promotes overall well-being. Stay creative, find activities you enjoy, and make staying active a natural part of your daily life.

Chapter 7

: Managing Hunger and Cravings

Managing hunger and cravings is an important aspect of a successful weight loss journey. Here are some strategies to help you effectively manage hunger and cravings:

Eat balanced meals: Ensure that your meals contain a balance of macronutrients (protein, carbohydrates, and healthy fats) as well as fiber-rich foods. This combination helps keep you feeling full and satisfied for longer periods.

Prioritize protein: Including protein-rich foods in your meals and snacks can help control hunger. Protein takes longer to digest and helps stabilize blood sugar levels, reducing the likelihood of cravings. Good sources of protein include lean meats, poultry, fish, tofu, legumes, and Greek yogurt.

Choose high-fiber foods: Foods high in fiber, such as fruits, vegetables, whole grains, and legumes, add bulk to your meals, promoting satiety. They also help regulate digestion and stabilize blood sugar levels, reducing cravings.

Ensure you stay well-hydrated: At times, we may confuse thirst for hunger. Maintain adequate hydration by drinking water consistently throughout the day. Drinking a glass of water before meals can also help reduce appetite. Opt for water over sugary beverages, which can contribute to increased cravings.

Plan and prepare meals: Plan your meals and snacks in advance, ensuring they are balanced and nutrient-dense. Having healthy options readily available can prevent impulsive choices or reaching for unhealthy snacks when hunger strikes.

Engage in mindful eating: Cultivate the habit of mindful eating by being aware of your body's signals of hunger and fullness. Take your time while eating, relish each bite, and heed your body's indications of satisfaction.

This helps you better recognize when you are genuinely hungry and when you are satisfied.

Include healthy fats: Incorporate sources of healthy fats, such as avocados, nuts, seeds, and olive oil, in your meals. Healthy fats provide satiety and help curb cravings. They also contribute to nutrient absorption and support overall health.

opt for whole foods: Choose whole, unprocessed foods over highly processed and sugary options. Whole foods are more nutrient-dense, satisfying, and better for your overall health. Processed foods can trigger cravings and lead to overeating.

Cope with stress effectively: Effectively managing stress is important as it can influence emotional eating patterns and cravings. Find healthy ways to manage stress, such as practicing relaxation techniques, engaging in physical activity, or seeking support from friends, family, or a counselor.

Get enough sleep: Inadequate sleep can disrupt hunger-regulating hormones, leading to increased appetite and cravings. Aim for 7-9 hours of quality sleep each night to support overall well-being and manage hunger effectively.

Distract yourself: When cravings strike, try distracting yourself with a non-food activity. Engage in a hobby, go for a walk, read a book, or call a friend. Redirecting your attention can help diminish cravings.

Embrace portion control: Stay mindful of the sizes of your portions and avoid overeating. Opt for smaller plates or bowls to give the illusion of a more satisfying meal. Pay attention to your body's cues of satisfaction and stop eating when you feel comfortably full.

Allow for occasional treats: It's important to allow yourself the occasional treat or indulgence. Completely depriving yourself of your favorite foods can lead to feelings of restriction and potential binge eating. Practice moderation and enjoy your favorite treats in controlled portions.

Remember, managing hunger and cravings is a journey, and it may take time to find what works best for you. Stay consistent with your healthy eating habits, be patient with yourself, and seek support from a registered dietitian or healthcare professional if needed

7.1 Strategies for Controlling Hunger

Controlling hunger is crucial when it comes to weight loss and maintaining a healthy diet. Here are some effective strategies for managing and controlling hunger:

Eat balanced meals: Opt for balanced meals that include a combination of protein, carbohydrates, and healthy fats. This helps provide sustained energy and keeps you feeling fuller for longer.

Prioritize protein: Protein-rich foods have been shown to promote feelings of fullness and reduce hunger. Include lean sources of protein such as chicken, fish, tofu, eggs, or legumes in your meals and snacks.

Include fiber-rich foods: Foods high in fiber, such as fruits, vegetables, whole grains, and legumes, add bulk to your meals and increase satiety. They also slow down digestion, helping you feel satisfied for a longer period.

Maintain proper hydration: Consume a sufficient quantity of water throughout the day. Sometimes, thirst can be mistaken for hunger. Before reaching for a snack, try drinking a glass of water and see if the hunger subsides.

Engage in mindful eating: Develop the habit of mindful eating by focusing your attention on the food, relishing each bite, and taking your time to eat slowly. This allows your brain to register feelings of fullness, preventing overeating.

Eat regular meals and snacks: Avoid skipping meals as it can lead to excessive hunger and overeating later on. Instead, aim to have regular meals and incorporate healthy snacks in between to keep your energy levels stable.

Opt for whole foods: Choose whole, unprocessed foods that are nutrient-dense and satisfying. These foods are often higher in fiber, protein, and essential nutrients, which can help control hunger.

Get enough sleep: Inadequate sleep has been linked to increased hunger and appetite. Aim for 7-9 hours of quality sleep per night to support your overall well-being and help regulate hunger hormones.

It is essential to effectively manage stress as it has the potential to induce emotional eating and stimulate cravings. Find healthy ways to manage stress, such as exercise, meditation, deep breathing, or engaging in hobbies that help you relax.

Include healthy fats: Healthy fats, such as avocados, nuts, seeds, and olive oil, provide satiety and help control hunger. Incorporate them into your meals and snacks to promote feelings of fullness.

Take the opportunity to thoroughly chew your food, ensuring that each bite is properly broken down before swallowing. Chewing not only aids in digestion but also allows your brain to register the act of eating, leading to a sense of satisfaction and fullness.

Use smaller plates and utensils: Serve your meals on smaller plates and use smaller utensils. This can create the illusion of a larger portion and help control portion sizes, preventing overeating.

Address emotional eating by seeking alternative methods to manage and cope with your emotions, rather than turning to food as a source of comfort or distraction. Engage in activities that help you relax, such as reading, listening to music, taking a walk, or talking to a supportive friend or family member.

Stay consistent with your eating routine: Try to establish regular meal and snack times. This helps regulate your hunger and satiety cues and prevents excessive hunger.

Remember that everyone's hunger and satiety levels are unique, so it's essential to listen to your body and adjust these strategies based on your individual needs. Consulting with a registered dietitian can also provide personalized guidance to help you control hunger and meet your weight loss goals

7.2 Dealing with Emotional Eating

Emotional eating refers to using food as a way to cope with or soothe emotions rather than as a response to physical hunger. It is a common behavior that can be challenging to overcome, but with the right strategies, you can develop healthier ways to deal with your emotions. Here are some strategies to help you manage emotional eating:

Identify the factors that tend to trigger emotional eating in order to develop awareness and better manage them.

Start by identifying the emotions or situations that tend to trigger your emotional eating. It could be stress, boredom, sadness, loneliness, or even certain social events. Increased self-awareness will help you anticipate and better manage these triggers.

Discover alternative strategies to manage your emotions rather than relying on food as a coping mechanism. Engage in activities that bring you joy and help you relax, such as practicing deep breathing, meditation, journaling, taking a walk, listening to music, or pursuing hobbies you enjoy.

Create a support system: Reach out to friends, family, or a support group who can offer understanding and encouragement during difficult times. Having someone to talk to can help you process your emotions and find healthier ways to address them.

Practice mindful eating: Develop a mindful eating practice to help you become more aware of your thoughts, emotions, and physical sensations related to eating. Be fully present and engage your senses while eating by paying close attention to the taste, texture, and aroma of your food. Eat slowly and savor each bite. This can help you distinguish between physical hunger and emotional cravings.

Keep a food and mood journal: Keep track of your food intake as well as your emotions and triggers in a journal. This can help you identify patterns and gain insight into your emotional eating habits. By recognizing the connections between your emotions and food choices, you can develop strategies to address them.

Create a healthy food environment: Surround yourself with nutritious food choices and remove or minimize the presence of trigger foods in your environment. Stock your pantry and refrigerator with healthy snacks and meals that align with your weight loss goals.

Practice stress management: Find healthy ways to manage stress, as stress can often trigger emotional eating. Engage in regular exercise, practice relaxation techniques such as deep breathing or meditation, and prioritize self-care activities that help you unwind.

If emotional eating is greatly affecting your life and impeding your efforts to maintain a healthy weight, it is advisable to seek support from a qualified professional. They can provide valuable guidance and assistance tailored to your specific situation, helping you address the underlying emotional triggers and develop healthier coping mechanisms. Remember, seeking help is a proactive step towards improving your well-being and achieving your weight management goals.

professional such as a therapist, counselor, or registered dietitian. They can provide specialized support and guidance tailored to your specific needs.

They can offer personalized guidance and support to address your individual needs.

Embrace self-kindness and cultivate a sense of compassion towards yourself as you embark on your weight loss journey. Remember that setbacks may happen, and it's okay to make mistakes. Treat yourself with kindness and understanding, focusing on progress rather than perfection.

Celebrate non-food victories: Shift your focus from using food as a reward or comfort to celebrating non-food victories. Recognize and celebrate achievements such as practicing self-care, engaging in physical activity, or reaching personal goals unrelated to food.

It's important to note that overcoming emotional eating takes time and patience. Be gentle with yourself as you navigate this process, and remember that you have the ability to develop healthier coping mechanisms that support both your emotional well-being and your weight loss goals.

7.3 Tips for Handling Food Cravings

Food cravings can be a challenge when trying to stick to a weight loss plan. Here are some tips to help you handle and manage food cravings effectively:

Understand the cause: Recognize that food cravings can stem from various factors, such as emotional triggers, nutrient deficiencies, hormonal changes, or habits. By understanding the underlying cause of your cravings, you can address them more effectively.

Distinguish between hunger and cravings: Pause and assess whether you are truly physically hungry or if it's a craving. Cravings are often specific and focused on certain foods, whereas physical hunger tends to be more general. If you're not genuinely hungry, it's likely a craving.

Practice mindful eating: Engage in mindful eating by slowing down and paying attention to your food choices and eating experience. Make a conscious effort to fully enjoy each bite, paying attention to the flavors and textures of the food, and tuning into your body's cues of hunger and fullness.

Adopting a mindful approach to eating can effectively reduce impulsive eating behaviors and enhance satisfaction, even when consuming smaller portions. By being fully present and attentive during meals, you become more aware of your body's hunger and fullness cues, allowing you to make conscious choices about what and how much you eat.

This increased mindfulness promotes a deeper appreciation of the eating experience, including the taste, texture, and aroma of food. Consequently, you can enhance your enjoyment of each mouthful, experience greater satiety, and reduce the inclination for impulsive eating.

By being fully present and attentive to the eating experience, you can better appreciate the flavors, textures, and satisfaction derived from each bite.

This can lead to a more balanced and mindful relationship with food, promoting healthier choices and portion control. Additionally, ensure adequate hydration by regularly drinking water, as dehydration can sometimes be mistaken for food cravings. When a craving strikes, have a glass of water first and see if it subsides.

Identify trigger foods: Take note of the foods that tend to trigger intense cravings for you. It could be certain types of sweets, salty snacks, or other indulgent treats. Be aware of these trigger foods and consider minimizing their presence in your environment.

Plan and prepare meals: Plan your meals and snacks in advance, ensuring they are balanced and satisfying. This helps reduce the likelihood of impulsive and unhealthy food choices when cravings arise. Make a committed effort to adhere to your meal plan to the best of your ability.

Choose healthier alternatives: If you're craving a specific food, look for healthier alternatives that can satisfy your taste buds. For example, if you're craving something sweet, opt for a piece of fruit or a small portion of dark chocolate instead of reaching for sugary treats.

Practice portion control: If you're craving a specific food, allow yourself to enjoy it in moderation. Practice portion control by having a small serving or sharing it with someone else. This allows you to satisfy the craving without derailing your progress.

Practice self-care: Take care of your overall well-being by engaging in self-care activities that help reduce stress and promote relaxation. This can include activities such as taking a bath, practicing yoga, meditating, or engaging in hobbies that bring you joy.

They can provide guidance and personalized If you find it difficult to manage persistent cravings, consider reaching out to a registered dietitian or healthcare professional for guidance and support. Strategies to help you navigate food cravings effectively.

Remember, cravings are a normal part of life, and occasional indulgences are okay. The key is to find a balance between satisfying your cravings in moderation and staying committed to your weight loss goals. Stay patient, be kind to yourself, and focus on the progress you're making toward a healthier lifestyle.

7.4 Mindful Eating and Portion Awareness

Mindful eating and portion awareness are two essential practices when it comes to maintaining a healthy diet and managing weight. Here's a breakdown of each concept and some tips to help you incorporate them into your daily routine:

Mindful Eating:

Mindful eating involves paying attention to your food, the sensations of eating, and your body's cues of hunger and fullness. By incorporating mindful eating into your routine, you can cultivate a healthier connection with food and make more intentional decisions. Here are some strategies to help you embrace mindful eating:

Slow down: Take your time to eat, savor each bite, and chew your food thoroughly. Eating slowly allows you to fully experience the flavors and textures of your food and promotes better digestion.

Eliminate distractions: Minimize distractions while eating, such as electronic devices or television. Instead, create a calm and peaceful environment where you can focus on your meal.

Engage your senses: Take notice of the colors, smells, and textures of your food. Be conscious of the flavors and sensations you experience while eating

Tune into hunger and fullness cues: Before you start eating, assess your hunger level on a scale of 1 to 10. Aim to eat when you're moderately hungry (around 3-4) and stop when you feel comfortably satisfied (around 6-7). Avoid eating until you're overly full.

Express gratitude: Prior to every meal, take a moment to acknowledge and appreciate the food in front of you. Developing a sense of gratitude can enhance your mindful eating experience and help you savor your meals.

Acknowledge emotional eating: Be aware of whether you are using food to manage emotions instead of responding to physical hunger. If you notice emotional eating patterns, explore alternative strategies to address your emotions, such as pursuing hobbies, seeking support from friends, or engaging in therapeutic activities like journaling.

Portion Awareness:

Portion awareness involves understanding appropriate serving sizes and controlling the amount of food you eat. It helps you maintain a balance between enjoying your favorite foods and managing calorie intake. Here are some tips for portion awareness:

Use measuring tools: Use measuring cups, spoons, or a kitchen scale to get familiar with proper portion sizes. This can help you accurately portion out foods until you develop a good eye for estimating serving sizes.

Fill your plate mindfully: When plating your meals, aim for a balance of vegetables, lean proteins, whole grains, and healthy fats. Visualize the recommended proportions of each food group on your plate to ensure a balanced meal.

Practice portion control strategies: If you're eating out or faced with large portions, consider using portion control strategies such as sharing a meal, ordering appetizer-sized portions, or requesting a to-go box to save leftovers.

Use smaller plates and bowls: Research suggests that using smaller plates and bowls can help you consume fewer calories without feeling deprived. The reduced plate size creates an optical illusion of a fuller plate, which can help you feel satisfied with less food.

Pay heed to your body: Be attentive to the cues of hunger and satiety that your body communicate. Eat until you feel comfortably satisfied, rather than clearing your plate or eating until you're overly full.

Focus on nutrient-dense foods: Prioritize nutrient-dense foods that offer high nutritional value in smaller portions. This way, you can feel satisfied while consuming fewer calories.

By practicing mindful eating and portion awareness, you can develop a better understanding of your body's needs, enjoy your meals more fully, and make choices that align with your weight loss goals. Remember, these practices take time and patience, so be kind to yourself as you incorporate them into your daily routine.

Chapter 8

Overcoming Weight Loss Plateaus

Weight loss plateaus are a common challenge that many people face during their weight loss journey. It can be frustrating and demotivating when your progress stalls, but there are strategies you can implement to overcome weight loss plateaus and continue making progress toward your goals. Here are some strategies to help you overcome a weight loss plateau:

Review your calorie intake: Assess your current calorie intake and ensure that you are still maintaining a calorie deficit. As you lose weight, your body's caloric needs may decrease, so adjusting your calorie intake accordingly can reignite weight loss. Consider tracking your food intake and using a food diary or mobile app to monitor your calories.

Mix up your exercise routine: If you've been following the same exercise routine for a while, your body may have adapted to it, resulting in a plateau. Add variety to your workouts by trying new exercises, increasing the intensity or duration of your workouts, or incorporating strength training to build muscle. Challenging your body in different ways can help stimulate weight loss.

Assess your portion sizes: Take a closer look at your portion sizes to ensure you're not unintentionally consuming more calories than you realize. It's easy to underestimate portion sizes, so consider using measuring cups, a food scale, or portion control containers to help you accurately portion your meals and snacks.

Reassess your goals: Take some time to revisit your weight loss goals and evaluate if they are realistic and attainable. Sometimes, adjusting your expectations and focusing on non-scale victories, such as improved energy levels or clothing fit, can provide a fresh perspective and renewed motivation.

Manage stress levels: High levels of stress can impact weight loss progress. Find healthy ways to manage stress, such as practicing relaxation techniques, engaging in physical activity, getting enough sleep, or seeking support from a therapist or counselor. By managing stress, you can support your overall well-being and potentially break through a weight loss plateau.

Get sufficient sleep: Inadequate sleep can disrupt hormone regulation and impact weight loss efforts. Strive to get between 7 to 9 hours of restful sleep per night to support your weight loss efforts. Establish a regular sleep schedule and optimize your sleep environment to enhance the quality and duration of your sleep.

Stay consistent and patient: Remember that weight loss plateaus are a normal part of the process. Stay committed to your healthy habits and remain patient. Weight loss is not always linear, and your body may need time to adjust. Trust the process and focus on making sustainable lifestyle changes rather than solely focusing on the number on the scale.

Seek support: If you're struggling to break through a weight loss plateau, consider seeking support from a registered dietitian, personal trainer, or weight loss support group. They can provide guidance, personalized strategies, and accountability to help you overcome the plateau and continue progressing toward your goals.

Remember, everyone's weight loss journey is unique, and plateaus are a common occurrence. By implementing these strategies, staying consistent, and maintaining a positive mindset, you can overcome weight loss plateaus and continue on the path to achieving your desired weight and overall well-being.

8.1 Understanding Plateaus

Plateaus are a common occurrence in various aspects of life, including weight loss journeys. When it comes to weight loss, a plateau refers to a period of time when your progress slows down or halts, and you experience little to no change in your body weight or measurements. Understanding plateaus is essential for managing expectations and staying motivated throughout your weight loss journey. Here are some key points to help you understand plateaus better:

Natural response of the body: Plateaus are a natural response of the body to changes in calorie intake and exercise routines. Initially, when you start a weight loss program, your body may respond quickly, leading to noticeable weight loss. However, over time, your body adapts to the changes, and your metabolism may adjust, resulting in a temporary stall in weight loss.

Physiological factors: Plateaus can be influenced by various physiological factors. As you lose weight, your body composition changes, and the rate at which you burn calories may decrease. Additionally, hormonal changes, such as fluctuations in thyroid function or cortisol levels, can impact your weight loss progress.

Loss of water weight: During the initial stages of weight loss, a significant portion of the weight you lose may come from water weight. This can make your progress seem more rapid in the beginning. However, once your body has shed excess water, further weight loss may occur at a slower pace, leading to a plateau.

Muscle gain: If you incorporate strength training or resistance exercises into your weight loss routine, you may experience an increase in muscle mass. While this is beneficial for your overall body composition, it can temporarily mask fat loss on the scale, creating the illusion of a plateau. Remember that muscle is denser than fat, so even if the scale doesn't change, you may still be making progress in terms of body composition.

Psychological factors: Plateaus can also have a psychological impact. When you're not seeing immediate results, it's easy to feel discouraged and lose motivation. It's important to understand that plateaus are a normal part of the process, and persistence is key to overcoming them.

Evaluation and adjustment: Plateaus provides an opportunity to reevaluate your approach and make necessary adjustments. Assess your current diet, exercise routine, and lifestyle habits. Look for areas where you can make positive changes, such as modifying your calorie intake, increasing your exercise intensity or duration, or trying new activities to challenge your body.

Non-scale victories: While the scale may not be moving, remember to focus on other signs of progress. Pay attention to how your clothes fit, changes in your energy levels, improved physical fitness, or positive changes in body measurements. Non-scale victories can be just as important and motivating as the number on the scale.

Patience and persistence: Plateaus can test your patience and resilience, but it's essential to stay positive and keep going. Keep in mind that weight loss occurs gradually, and long-term success relies on maintaining consistency and commitment. Trust the process, stay committed to your healthy habits, and have confidence that progress will resume.

By understanding plateaus as a natural part of the weight loss journey, you can better navigate through them without feeling discouraged. Embrace the opportunity to reassess your approach, stay patient, and focus on the overall progress you're making toward a healthier lifestyle.

8.2 Analyzing Your Progress

Analyzing your progress is a crucial step in any weight loss journey. It allows you to assess how far you've come, identify areas of improvement, and make necessary adjustments to keep moving forward. Here are some key factors to consider when analyzing your progress:

Regular weigh-ins: Weighing yourself regularly can provide a quantitative measurement of your progress. However, it's important to keep in mind that weight can fluctuate due to various factors such as water retention, hormonal changes, or muscle gain. Instead of focusing solely on the number on the scale, consider trends over time and track your weight in conjunction with other indicators of progress.

Body measurements: Taking body measurements can provide a more comprehensive picture of your progress. Measure areas such as your waist, hips, thighs, and arms. As you lose body fat, you may notice changes in these measurements, even if the scale doesn't show significant changes. Record your measurements regularly to track your progress accurately.

Body composition analysis: Consider getting a body composition analysis done, either through a professional assessment or with the help of smart scales or handheld devices. This analysis provides insights into your body fat percentage, muscle mass, and other valuable metrics. It helps you track changes in body composition, which is a better indicator of progress than weight alone.

Fitness assessments: Assessing your fitness levels can give you an idea of how your physical fitness is improving. Keep track of parameters such as cardiovascular endurance, strength, flexibility, and balance. Set benchmarks and periodically evaluate your performance to see if there's any progress.

Be mindful of your energy levels and mood throughout the day, and take note of any fluctuations or patterns. Are you experiencing increased energy levels, improved sleep quality, and enhanced mood? These subjective indicators can reflect positive changes in your overall well-being and are valuable signs of progress.

Clothing fit: Notice how your clothes fit and if you need to adjust sizes or if there are noticeable changes in how they feel on your body. Looser-fitting clothes or needing to tighten belts can be indications of body composition changes, regardless of what the scale says.

Non-scale victories: Celebrate non-scale victories, such as achieving personal fitness milestones, making healthier food choices, overcoming cravings, or sticking to your exercise routine consistently. These small victories are important markers of progress and can boost your motivation.

Self-reflection and self-assessment: Take the time to reflect on your journey and assess how you're feeling both physically and mentally. Are you feeling more confident, motivated, and empowered? Are you developing healthier habits and a more positive relationship with food and exercise? Personal growth and positive mindset shifts are vital aspects of progress.

Remember that progress is not always linear, and there may be ups and downs along the way. Embrace the journey as a whole and look for overall improvements rather than getting fixated on immediate results. Regularly analyzing your progress allows you to make informed decisions, stay motivated, and adjust your strategies as needed to achieve long-term success in your weight loss journey.

8.3 Adjusting Your Diet and Exercise

Adjusting your diet and exercise is a critical aspect of a successful weight loss journey. As you progress, your body may adapt to your initial changes, and you might reach a point where further adjustments are needed to continue making progress toward your weight loss goals. Here are some key considerations for adjusting your diet and exercise:

Reassess your calorie intake: As you lose weight, your caloric needs may change. It's essential to reassess your calorie intake periodically to ensure you're still in a calorie deficit. Consider consulting a registered dietitian or using online calculators to determine your current calorie needs based on your updated weight, activity level, and goals. Adjust your calorie intake accordingly to continue losing weight at a healthy and sustainable rate.

Fine-tune your macronutrient ratios: While creating a calorie deficit is crucial for weight loss, the distribution of macronutrients (carbohydrates, proteins, and fats) in your diet can also impact your results. Evaluate your macronutrient ratios and consider adjusting them based on your individual needs and preferences. For example, you may find that increasing protein intake helps you feel fuller and preserves lean muscle mass, while adjusting carbohydrate and fat intake provides the energy you need for workouts.

Modify meal timing and frequency: Experiment with meal timing and frequency to find a pattern that works best for you. Some individuals may prefer three balanced meals per day, while others might thrive with smaller, more frequent meals or intermittent fasting. Find a schedule that suits your lifestyle and helps you maintain a calorie deficit without feeling overly restricted or deprived.

Increase exercise intensity or duration: If your weight loss has slowed down, consider increasing the intensity or duration of your workouts. Challenge yourself with higher resistance in strength training exercises, increase the speed or incline on cardio workouts, or add extra sets and repetitions to your routines. Progressive overload, where you gradually increase the demands on your body, can help stimulate further weight loss and prevent plateaus.

Incorporate new exercises: Shake up your exercise routine by incorporating new activities or exercises. Trying different workouts not only prevents boredom but also challenges your body in different ways. Consider adding activities such as high-intensity interval training (HIIT), yoga, Pilates, swimming, or cycling to diversify your workouts and engage different muscle groups.

Seek professional guidance: If you're unsure about how to adjust your diet or exercise routine, consider consulting with a registered dietitian or certified personal trainer. They can provide personalized guidance based on your individual needs, preferences, and goals. They will assess your current plan, make recommendations, and help you create a sustainable and effective approach for continued progress.

Listen to your body: Pay attention to how your body responds to changes in diet and exercise. Each individual is unique, and what may be effective for one person may not necessarily be the same for someone else. Be mindful of any signs of overexertion, fatigue, or excessive hunger. Adjust your approach based on how your body feels and find a balance that promotes both weight loss and overall well-being.

Remember that making adjustments is a normal part of the weight loss process. Give yourself time and have faith in the process Give yourself time and have faith in the process. It's important to focus on sustainable changes that promote long-term health and well-being. By continually assessing and adjusting your diet and exercise, you can overcome plateaus, keep progressing, and achieve your weight loss goals.

8.4 Seeking Support and Accountability

Seeking support and accountability is a powerful strategy for maintaining motivation and staying on track with your weight loss goals. When you have a strong support system and external accountability, it becomes easier to overcome challenges, stay consistent, and celebrate your successes. Here are some suggestions for finding support and maintaining accountability:

Find a weight loss buddy: Partnering up with someone who shares similar goals can provide tremendous support and accountability. Look for a friend, family member, or colleague who is also on a weight loss journey or interested in adopting a healthier lifestyle. You can share your experiences, challenges, and successes, and hold each other accountable for sticking to your goals.

Join a support group: Participating in a weight loss support group or online community can provide a sense of camaraderie and understanding. These groups offer a safe space to share your struggles, seek advice, and celebrate milestones with individuals who are going through similar experiences. Engage actively in discussions, offer support to others, and draw inspiration from their stories.

Enlist the help of a professional: Consider working with a registered dietitian, certified personal trainer, or weight loss coach who can provide expert guidance and support. These professionals can design personalized meal plans, create exercise routines tailored to your needs, and offer valuable advice to keep you motivated and accountable. They can also track your progress, provide feedback, and make necessary adjustments along the way.

Share your goals with loved ones: Openly communicate your weight loss goals with your close friends, family, or significant other. Their support, motivation, and empathy can have a meaningful impact on your path to success. Stay focused, and offer assistance when needed.

Utilize technology and apps: There are numerous apps and online tools available that can assist you in tracking your progress and providing accountability. These apps can help you monitor your calorie intake, track your exercise routines, set reminders, and even connect with like-minded individuals for added support. Discover various alternatives and identify the ones that align with your specific needs and preferences.

Celebrate milestones: Celebrating your achievements, no matter how small, is crucial for maintaining motivation. When you reach a milestone or accomplish a goal, take time to acknowledge your success and reward yourself in a non-food-related way. This positive reinforcement reinforces your progress and encourages you to keep moving forward.

Track your progress: Keep a record of your journey, including your weight, measurements, fitness achievements, and other relevant markers of progress. Regularly reviewing your progress can provide a visual representation of how far you've come and motivate you to keep pushing forward.

Be accountable to yourself: While external support is valuable, self-accountability is equally important. Set clear, realistic goals for yourself, establish a routine, and hold yourself responsible for sticking to your plan. Practice self-discipline and cultivate a positive mindset to overcome obstacles and stay committed to your weight loss journey.

Remember, seeking support and accountability is not a sign of weakness but a smart strategy for success. Surrounding yourself with people who uplift and encourage you, while also holding you accountable, can greatly enhance your chances of reaching your weight loss goals. Embrace the power of community, be open to help, and stay committed to your journey.

Chapter 9

Maintaining Weight Loss

Sustaining weight loss is equally crucial to accomplishing it. after putting in the effort to lose weight, you want to ensure that you can sustain your progress and prevent regaining the weight. Here are several fundamental approaches to sustaining weight loss:

Maintain a balanced and nutritious diet: Continue to prioritize a balanced diet rich in whole foods, lean proteins, fruits, vegetables, and healthy fats. Pay attention to the size of your servings and adopt a moderate approach to eating. Avoid drastic restrictions or overly restrictive diets that are not sustainable in the long term. Aim for consistency rather than perfection.

Stay physically active: Regular exercise is crucial for maintaining weight loss and overall health. Discover activities that bring you joy and incorporate them into your regular schedule. Refrain from participating in unconscious eating, relying on food as an emotional crutch, or giving in to eating out of sheer boredom. Stay consistent with your exercise regimen, but also listen to your body and give it proper rest and recovery.

Set realistic goals: While it's essential to have goals, be mindful of setting realistic and sustainable ones. Avoid setting unrealistic goals for weight or body size that may be challenging to sustain in the long term. Focus on overall well-being, health, and strength rather than just the number on the scale. Celebrate non-scale victories and the positive changes you've made in your lifestyle.

Steer clear of setting unattainable goals for weight or body size that may be difficult to maintain over the long run. It helps with digestion, keeps you hydrated, and can contribute to a feeling of fullness. Drink an adequate amount of water throughout the day and limit sugary drinks or excessive alcohol consumption.

Make sleep a priority: Getting sufficient sleep is essential for weight management. Inadequate sleep can disturb hunger and fullness hormones, resulting in heightened cravings and overeating. Strive for 7-8 hours of restful sleep each night to help maintain a healthy weight.

Monitor your progress: Regularly assess your weight, measurements, and body composition to stay aware of any changes. If you notice any significant fluctuations, reflect on your habits and make necessary adjustments. Regular monitoring can help you catch any potential regain early on and take action to address it.

Stay accountable and seek support: Continue to seek support and accountability from friends, family, or online communities that share your health and weight loss goals. Consider joining maintenance-focused groups or programs where you can connect with others who are also working to maintain their weight loss. Stay accountable to yourself by tracking your food intake, exercise, and progress.

Be flexible and adapt: Life is full of ups and downs, and your weight may fluctuate due to various factors such as stress, hormonal changes, or special occasions. Embrace flexibility in your approach and learn to adapt to different situations. If you have a setback, don't be too hard on yourself. Instead, focus on getting back on track and maintaining a healthy balance.

Keep in mind that sustaining weight loss is an ongoing process that spans a lifetime. Be patient, kind to yourself, and un Make sleep a priority: Getting sufficient sleep is essential for weight management. Inadequate sleep can disturb hunger and fullness hormones, resulting in heightened cravings and overeating. Strive for 7-8 hours of restful sleep each night to help maintain a healthy weight. Focus on sustainable habits, prioritize your health, and celebrate the progress you've made. By adopting a balanced and mindful approach, you can successfully maintain your weight loss and enjoy a healthier and happier life.

9.1 Strategies for Long-Term Success

Achieving long-term success with weight loss requires adopting strategies that promote sustainable habits and a healthy lifestyle. Here are some effective strategies to help you maintain your weight loss and achieve long-term success:

Set realistic and achievable goals: Set realistic weight loss goals and break them down into smaller milestones. By doing so, you can monitor your progress and maintain your motivation. Avoid setting overly ambitious targets that may be difficult to maintain in the long run.

Focus on sustainable lifestyle changes: Instead of relying on short-term diets or extreme measures, focus on making sustainable lifestyle changes. Gradually incorporate healthy eating habits, regular exercise, and positive behavior changes into your daily routine. This approach ensures that your weight loss efforts are sustainable and can be maintained over time.

Build a balanced and varied diet: Incorporate a wide variety of fruits, vegetables, whole grains, lean proteins, and healthy fats into your diet. Strive for balance and moderation, and limit the consumption of processed foods, sugary drinks, and snacks high in saturated fats and added sugars.

Stay physically active: Regular exercise is crucial for maintaining weight loss. Incorporate activities that bring you joy into your regular routine. Strive for a balanced fitness regimen that includes a mix of cardiovascular exercises, strength training, and flexibility exercises. Consistency is key, so find ways to stay motivated and make exercise a priority.

Practice mindful eating: Be present and conscious of your eating habits. Take your time while eating, fully enjoy each bite, and be mindful of your body's cues for hunger and fullness. Minimize distractions like television or electronic devices, as they can lead to overeating.

Manage stress in an effective manner: Acknowledge that stress can impact emotional eating and create barriers to reaching your weight loss objectives. Find healthy ways to manage stress, such as practicing relaxation techniques, engaging in physical activity, getting enough sleep, and seeking support from loved ones or professionals when needed.

Maintain proper hydration: Ensure you consume an adequate amount of water throughout the day to stay properly hydrated. Water can help control appetite, support digestion, and keep you energized. Limit the consumption of sugary beverages and alcohol, as they can contribute to excess calorie intake.

Regularly monitor and adjust your habits: Keep track of your progress, including weight, measurements, and body composition. Regularly assess your eating and exercise habits to identify areas for improvement. If you notice any weight fluctuations, be proactive in adjusting your behaviors to get back on track.

Seek support and accountability: Surround yourself with a supportive network of friends, family, or a weight loss community. Engage in open communication with them, sharing your goals, challenges, and achievements.

Seek professional assistance: Consider seeking guidance from a registered dietitian, or personal trainer, or joining a weight loss support group to receive expert advice, stay motivated, and remain accountable.

Celebrate your milestones: Take the time to acknowledge and appreciate your achievements, no matter how small they may be. Recognize the progress you have made and use it as a source of motivation to continue on your weight loss journey. Reward yourself with non-food-related treats, such as a Consider treating yourself to a massage, purchasing new workout attire, or taking a well-deserved day off to unwind and recharge.

Remember, maintaining weight loss is a lifelong journey that requires consistency, dedication, and a positive mindset. Embrace a sustainable approach, be patient with yourself, and focus on creating a healthy and balanced lifestyle that supports long-term success.

9.2 Building Healthy Habits

Building healthy habits is a crucial component of long-term success in weight loss and overall well-being. By focusing on developing sustainable habits, you can create a foundation for a healthier lifestyle. Here are some strategies to help you build and maintain healthy habits:

Start with small, achievable changes: Begin by making small, manageable changes to your daily routine. This could involve incorporating more fruits and vegetables into your meals, swapping sugary beverages for water, or taking a short walk after dinner. Progressively elevate the difficulty or intensity of your routines as you go along.

Establish well-defined and quantifiable objectives: Clearly outline your goals to establish a sense of direction and inspiration. Ensure your goals are attainable, measurable, specific, relevant, and time-bound. For example, aim to eat five servings of vegetables per day or exercise for 30 minutes five days a week. Tracking your progress can help you stay accountable and celebrate achievements.

Establishing a routine is essential for developing consistent habits. Establish a regular routine by scheduling dedicated time for exercise, meal planning, and self-care. By incorporating these activities into your daily or weekly schedule, they become a natural part of your lifestyle.

Identify and overcome obstacles: Recognize the obstacles that may hinder your progress and develop strategies to overcome them. For example, if time constraints make it difficult to cook healthy meals, consider meal prepping on weekends or finding quick and nutritious recipes. Anticipating and addressing potential challenges can help you stay on track.

Make self-care a priority: Give importance to activities that prioritize your physical, mental, and emotional well-being. This could include getting enough sleep, managing stress through relaxation techniques or hobbies, engaging in activities you enjoy, and taking time for yourself. When you prioritize self-care, you're better equipped to make healthy choices and maintain positive habits.

Focus on progress, not perfection: Building healthy habits is a process, and it's important to embrace the journey. Recognize that setbacks and slip-ups are normal and part of the learning process. Instead of aiming for perfection, focus on progress and celebrate each step forward, no matter how small.

9.3 Managing Weight Maintenance Challenges

Maintaining weight loss can come with its own set of challenges, but with the right strategies and mindset, you can overcome them. Here are some tips for managing weight maintenance challenges:

Stay consistent with healthy habits: Consistency is key in weight maintenance. Continue practicing the healthy habits you adopted during your weight loss journey, such as regular exercise, portion control, and making nutritious food choices. Don't view weight maintenance as a destination but rather as an ongoing process of sustaining healthy habits.

Monitor your progress: Regularly track your weight, measurements, and other relevant markers to stay aware of any changes. Monitoring your progress can help you catch any potential weight regain early on and make necessary adjustments to your lifestyle. Remember that weight fluctuations are normal, and focus on overall trends rather than day-to-day changes.

Maintain awareness of your eating habits: Continue incorporating mindful eating into your routine by being attentive to your body's hunger and fullness signals, taking your time to eat slowly, and appreciating each bite. Remain watchful for triggers that may lead to emotional eating and actively seek out alternative strategies to effectively manage stress or emotions. Stay present while eating and enjoy the experience.

Find new sources of motivation: Keep your motivation high by finding new sources of inspiration. Set new goals that go beyond the number on the scale, such as improving fitness levels, participating in a charity run, or trying new physical activities. Celebrate non-scale victories, like increased energy, improved sleep quality, or enhanced mood.

Plan for challenging situations: Anticipate challenging situations such as social events, holidays, or vacations, and plan accordingly. Have strategies in place to navigate these situations, such as choosing healthier options, practicing portion control, or engaging in physical activities during vacations. Remember that occasional indulgences are part of a balanced lifestyle, but be mindful of your choices.

Be flexible and adaptable: Recognize that your weight may fluctuate naturally due to factors like water retention, hormonal changes, or variations in muscle mass. Be flexible and adapt to changes by making adjustments to your eating and exercise routine as needed. Embrace the mindset of lifelong learning and adjust your approach based on your evolving needs.

Remember, weight maintenance is a lifelong journey. Embrace the challenges you encounter as valuable opportunities for personal growth and learning. Focus on sustainable habits, self-care, and finding joy in a healthy lifestyle. With perseverance and a positive mindset, you can overcome weight maintenance challenges and enjoy the benefits of long-term success.

Conclusion

In conclusion, understanding weight loss is essential for embarking on a successful journey toward a healthier lifestyle. It involves recognizing the factors that affect weight loss, setting realistic goals, assessing your current state, and making changes to your habits and behaviors.

By understanding the importance of nutrition, macronutrients, portion control, and incorporating nutrient-dense foods into your diet, you can create a balanced and effective weight loss plan. Additionally, incorporating exercise, staying hydrated, and managing hunger and cravings play vital roles in achieving your weight loss goals.

Throughout your weight loss journey, it is crucial to stay motivated, seek support, and celebrate your achievements. Building healthy habits, overcoming obstacles, and developing strategies for long-term success are key elements in maintaining your weight loss.

Remember, weight loss is a personal journey, and it is important to listen to your body, make sustainable choices, and be patient with yourself. Embrace the process of self-discovery, learning, and growth. By implementing the knowledge and strategies outlined in this guide, you can make positive changes in your life and achieve your weight loss goals.

Appendix A: Grocery Shopping List

When embarking on a weight loss journey, having a well-planned grocery shopping list can be a valuable tool to help you make healthier choices and stay on track with your goals. Here's a sample grocery shopping list that includes a variety of nutritious foods:

Fruits and vegetables:

Apple

Berries (strawberries, blueberries, raspberries)

Bananas

Oranges

Spinach

Broccoli

Cauliflower

Carrots

Bell peppers

Tomatoes

Whole grains and cereals:

Whole wheat bread

Brown rice

Quinoa

Oats

Whole grain pasta

Whole grain cereal

Lean proteins:

Skinless chicken breast

Turkey breast

Fish (salmon, cod, tuna)

Lean cuts of beef (sirloin, tenderloin)

Eggs

Greek yogurt

Cottage cheese

Plant-based protein sources (tofu, lentils, beans)

Dairy or dairy alternatives:

Skim milk

Greek yogurt (plain, unsweetened)

Low-fat cheese

Almond milk or other non-dairy milk alternatives

Healthy fats:

Avocados

Olive oil

Nuts (almonds, walnuts, cashews)

Seeds (chia seeds, flaxseeds)

Legumes and beans:

Chickpeas

Black beans

Lentils

Condiments and spices

Herbs and spices (oregano, basil, cinnamon, turmeric)

Low-sodium soy sauce

Hot sauce

Mustard

Salsa

Balsamic vinegar

Olive oil-based salad dressings (choose low-fat options)

Snacks and treats (in moderation):

Air-popped popcorn

Rice cakes

Dark chocolate (70% cocoa or higher)

Nut butter (almond butter, peanut butter)

Dried fruits (unsweetened)

Hydration:

Water

Herbal teas

Sparkling water (unsweetened)

Remember, this is just a sample grocery shopping list to get you started. Customize it based on your personal preferences, dietary restrictions, and specific weight loss plan. Be mindful of portion sizes and prioritize fresh, whole foods over processed options. Don't forget to check your pantry and fridge before shopping to avoid buying duplicate items.

Happy and healthy grocery shopping!